THE
metabolism
ADVANTAGE

An 8-Week Program to
Rev Up Your Body's
Fat-Burning Machine—**At Any Age**

THE
metabolism
ADVANTAGE

John Berardi, PhD, CSCS

RODALE

© 2006 by John Berardi

Photographs © 2006 by Rodale Inc.

Rodale books may be purchased for business or promotional use or for special sales. For information, please write to: Special Markets Department, Rodale, Inc., 733 Third Avenue, New York, NY 10017

Printed in the United States of America

Rodale Inc. makes every effort to use acid-free ∞, recycled paper ♻.

Library of Congress Cataloging-in-Publication Data

Berardi, John.
  The metabolism advantage : an 8-week program to rev up your body's fat-burning machine–at any age / John Berardi.
      p.   cm.
  Includes index.
  ISBN-13 978-1-59486-323-3 trade hardcover
  ISBN-10 1-59486-323-7 trade hardcover
  1. Weight loss.   2. Reducing diets.   3. Metabolism.   4. Nutrition.
5. Exercise.   I. Title.
  RM222.2.B446 2006
  613.2'5—dc22   2006018552

Distributed to the book trade by Holtzbrinck Publishers

We inspire and enable people to improve their lives and the world around them

For more of our products visit **rodalestore.com** or call 800-848-4735

Contents

Acknowledgments

In the book *Every Second Counts*, Lance Armstrong and Sally Jenkins note that "anyone who imagines they can work alone winds up surrounded by nothing but rivals, without companions. The fact is, no one ascends alone."

In the case of this book, never was a truer statement put forth. Without the expertise, insight, hospitality, care, support, friendship, and good humor of a virtual army of generous clients, colleagues, and friends, there would have been no ascent—and, of course, there would have been no *The Metabolism Advantage*. For all of their contributions to me personally and professionally, I'd like to acknowledge the following individuals for helping to make *The Metabolism Advantage* a reality.

To my good friends and Science Link partners, Phil Caravaggio and Carter Schoffer, it's been quite a ride! Don't for a second doubt that without you there would be no Science Link, no JohnBerardi. com, no Gourmet Nutrition, no *Scrawny to Brawny*, and no *The Metabolism Advantage*. Certainly don't doubt the fact that without you the thousands of people we've touched would have remained confused within the minefield of today's health, nutrition, and fitness "industries." In fact, don't even doubt that without you I wouldn't be in a white padded room rocking back and forth right now.

John Lennon said, "I get by with a little help from my friends." Me, I get by with *a lot* of help from my friends. Thanks for picking up the slack when there was some to pick up, thanks for lending ideas when mine had dried up, thanks for providing encouragement when I've been ready to give up. Thank you also for being ever-present examples of dedication, discipline, integrity, and uncompromising quality. They say that the company we keep determines who we'll be in the future. If this is true, the future looks bright indeed.

To the amazing clients of Science Link, my warmest thanks for becoming the very platform from which books like this can be created. Without your trust in our methods and systems, without your patience, and without your appreciation for the process of trial and error that accompanies the consulting relationship, translating research into real, measurable, and teachable results would never have come so easy. This book springs forth from your own successes and is just as much yours as it is mine.

To my colleagues at Rodale Inc.—without your support of my ideas, confidence in my writing, and faith in my ability to help people change the way they live, books like this would not be available to help so many. Thanks for making my vision a reality.

Finally, I'd like to acknowledge the researchers who've made it their life's work to uncover the mysteries of the human body. As Isaac Newton once said, "If I have seen further, it's only because I've stood on the shoulders of giants." To the aforementioned researchers, it is upon your shoulders I stand. Without your countless hours in the lab, I'd have no advice to give—this book is a tribute to your efforts.

PART 1

METABOLISM ADVANTAGE SCIENCE

Introduction

Even you can burn 40 to 60 percent more calories in 8 short weeks!

I remember the day I got the bad news. I was 20 years old, and I was in the middle of a great leg workout. I was breathing hard and resting between sets when an "older" personal trainer (he was probably in his thirties) came over and offered some "advice"—unsolicited, of course.

"Ya know," he said, "I used to look like you. Just you wait. After 25, the metabolism slows down, and it's all downhill from there, buddy. You'd better enjoy it while it lasts." Then he turned and walked away.

I wasn't sure what to make of this guy. After all, he didn't look that great. Sure, he was a trainer, and he did look better than most folks his age, but just barely. And he had a lot less muscle and a lot more fat than I did.

So I wondered if he was right. Does metabolism come to a grinding halt after age 25? Was I doomed to lose the youthful body that I was working so hard to develop?

I had to find out. After all, if middle-age spread is an inevitable consequence of aging, why bother? Why work so hard to maintain this fit, hard body? I might as well just throw in the towel right then.

So I asked around. I spoke with personal trainers, gym owners, and nutritionists, who all confirmed what I had heard. I talked to some instructors at my local community college. They said the same, although with less certainty, since at that time, not much research had been done on the subject.

I looked around, studying the physiques of people I ran into at the gym, grocery store, mall, and elsewhere. The evidence was all around me: Younger people were leaner and seemingly had faster metabolic rates than older folks.

Thus, in my 20-year-old mind, the message seemed clear: I'd better make the most of my youthful body and metabolism, because I was destined to lose it.

Fortunately, I was dead wrong! (And, I might add, so were the trainers, nutritionists, and university instructors I had consulted.)

Deceiving Father Time

Since that day, I've accomplished quite a bit in the exercise, nutrition, and fitness realm. I've spent 10 more years in school, earning a PhD in the area of exercise and nutritional biochemistry. I also developed an exercise and nutrition consulting company called Science Link, with the mission of taking advanced exercise and nutrition research and translating it into meaningful, usable information for people who aren't quite as science-minded as I am. During this time, I've had the opportunity to consult with thousands of individuals—from soccer stars to soccer coaches to soccer moms—and help them improve their health, body composition, performance, and metabolism.

Now in my thirties, I'm just as active as ever and, interestingly, just as fit, strong, and lean as I was during my twenties. I'm happy to report that metabolism *does not* have to slow down with age. Yes, it's true that when you're young, your body finds a way to balance energy expenditure and energy intake. It's true that as you age, you'll have a much more difficult time maintaining your healthiest body weight. It's true that studies have shown that one-third of all North American adults are at least 20 percent over their "ideal weights."

These truths, however, don't seal your fate. Just because some folks spend their lives engaged in a frustrating cycle of eating less only to gain more, that doesn't mean *you* have to. I've skirted around those so-called truths. I eat just as much food as I did in my twenties—if not more—yet I have no more body fat to show for it.

I'm not an anomaly. Over the years, I've trained countless clients, ranging in age from 25 to 65. It didn't matter how high their body fat percentages, how slow their metabolisms, or how scrawny their muscle mass when they met me—they were all able to turn things around, restoring the metabolism of their twenties. Consider the following impressive stats.

- Robert, age 41: Lost 18 pounds of fat and gained 8 pounds of lean mass (lean mass is made up of muscle, bone, and other non-fat tissue) over 3 months
- Kenneth, age 31: Lost 27 pounds of fat and gained 2 pounds of lean mass over 6 months
- Lynn, age 57: Lost 24 pounds of fat and gained 8 pounds of lean mass over 7 months
- Danielle, age 32: Lost 14 pounds of fat and gained 17 pounds of lean mass over 5 months
- Ben, age 21: Lost 14 pounds of fat and gained 29 pounds of lean mass over 10 months
- Gail, age 26: Lost 9 pounds of fat and gained 6 pounds of lean mass over 2 months
- Jason, age 45: Lost 11 pounds of fat and gained 3 pounds of lean mass over 3 months
- Kelly, age 38: Lost 22 pounds of fat and gained 15 pounds of lean mass over 6 months

- Mike, age 26: Lost 12 pounds of fat and gained 11 pounds of lean mass over 2 months
- Rachel, age 24: Lost 23 pounds of fat and gained 3 pounds of lean mass over 7 months
- Vivian, age 38: Lost 15 pounds of fat and gained 8 pounds of lean mass over 5 months
- Amy, age 38: Lost 29 pounds of fat and gained 10 pounds of lean mass over 9 months
- Joseph, age 42: Lost 4 pounds of fat and gained 38 pounds of lean mass over 13 months

As you can see, it doesn't matter how old people were when they decided to get serious and turn things around. Whether they were 25 or 45, their results were the same: They changed their body composition, replacing flab with lean, metabolism-boosting muscle. You're never too old to boost your metabolism.

Ian, one of my favorite clients, is living proof. Throughout his life, he had tried to stay fit and eat the right foods. But when he came to me at age 55, he admitted that he seemed to be fighting a losing battle. With each year, his gut seemed to grow a bit larger and his muscles somewhat smaller. When Ian started my program in February of 2005, he weighed 217 pounds and had 18 percent body fat. Within 6 months, he had shed 9 pounds of fat. "At my age, I had become a little too stuffy in my thinking about what I could and could not do in the gym," he told me. "You taught me to dispel that notion. I never would have thought that I would be doing split squats, sumo deadlifts, scarecrows, and the like. More important, my body has really changed. My fiancée has no problem walking with me on the beach (with my shirt off) by the volleyball courts, where all the hunks tend to hang out."

If that's not enough to convince you that you have what it takes to rev up your metabolism, shed fat, and build muscle, then consider the research. When I was in my twenties, few scientists had tried to answer the questions that were nagging me. At that time, no one really knew for sure whether metabolism slowed down with age or, if it did, whether anything could be done about it. Now a group of applied scientists have looked at those questions and uncovered some surprising facts.

These scientists had noticed that metabolism does seem to slow with age, but they refused to believe that there was nothing anyone could do about it. Today, as a result of their efforts, we've got plenty of evidence demonstrating that your metabolism slows with age *only if you do nothing about it*. If you eat properly, exercise, and take the right supplements, you can maintain your metabolic rate over your life span! Even if you're 40 or older and things have already slowed down, you can reverse the trend and regain the metabolism of your youth. In fact, you can create a metabolism that's even faster than the one you had your twenties!

Is it easy? No. Does it take hard work and dedication? Yes. But it can be done. I'm living proof. So are my clients, and so are the thousands of people who have participated in hundreds of studies conducted in the United States and around the world.

Of Age and Metabolism

So why does maintaining a healthy weight get tougher as we age? Well, although most people eat less as they age—to compensate for moving less at their desk jobs—their activity levels generally decrease even more than their energy intakes, resulting in fat gain.

These decreasing activity levels result in yet another problem: muscle loss. Researchers have determined that, starting between the ages of 25 and 30, most people lose roughly 5 to 10 pounds of muscle during each decade of life. Muscle is a metabolically active tissue, which means that in addition to burning calories to move your skeleton through space, it also burns calories to maintain itself. Thus, age-related muscle loss can cripple your metabolism. The average person who becomes less active and consequently loses muscle experiences a

20 to 25 percent reduction in 24-hour metabolism (measured as the amount of energy your body burns in 24 hours) by age 65. This adds up to a daily metabolic drop of more than 500 calories. Since it's tough to cut 500 calories from your daily menu to compensate for that metabolic drop, most people end up packing on the fat.

Of course, this scenario holds true only if you do nothing to prevent it. Why do most people lose muscle as they age? Because they don't use it. When it comes to the human body, what you don't use, you lose, and muscle is no exception.

Studies of people over age 60 show that you can—at any age—reverse muscle loss and regain the metabolism of your youth. In fact, according to research, individuals who—through exercise and smart eating—maintain their lean mass as they age experience only a 0.36 percent drop in metabolism per decade instead of the 5 to 7 percent drop that most adults experience. Add a few key supplements to the mix, and you can even prevent that 0.36 percent drop—and possibly even rev your metabolism higher than it was during your youth!

So metabolic slowdown is not inevitable. You can prevent it. And you can reverse it. *The Metabolism Advantage* will show you how.

The Metabolism Advantage approach is a three-pronged system for restoring the metabolism of your youth. It includes eating, exercising, and supplementing. With a nutritional plan that prioritizes metabolically costly proteins, metabolism-boosting fats, antioxidant-rich fruits and veggies, and the right carbs at the right times, *The Metabolism Advantage* will teach you how to stoke your metabolic fire in order to create a body and vitality that 20-year-olds will envy.

With a unique and individualized combination of interval exercise and strength training, you can further fire your metabolism. Finally, with the right supplement program, one containing specific nutrients that you simply can't get enough of from foods alone, *The Metabolism Advantage* will help you supercharge your metabolic engine and ensure that the new body you build today will put your previous best to shame.

Follow this time-tested, research-proven Metabolism Advantage program, and you'll soon find yourself in the best shape of your life. On the Metabolism Advantage plan, you will:

- **Build the muscle needed to speed up your resting metabolism all day and all night long.** The 5 to 10 pounds of lean mass muscle you can expect to build during the next 8 to 16 weeks will rev up your resting metabolism—the number of calories your body burns to maintain life—by roughly 100 calories.

- **Maximize something called the afterburn.** Through targeted strength training and cardio workouts, you'll increase not only the number of calories you burn during your workouts (about 300 to 600 calories per day, depending on your body size and workout duration) but also the calories you burn after your workouts (another 100 to 200 calories per day). These workouts will increase the number of calories your body uses to repair muscle tissue, replace nutrients, and otherwise recover from intense exercise.

- **Increase the number of calories your body burns as it digests foods** (another 100 to 200 calories per day).

- **Encourage your body to waste calories.** The foods and supplements you'll consume on the Metabolism Advantage plan will make your body a much less efficient calorie burner. Much like a car in need of a tune-up, your body will consume more fuel than it needs to operate, eliminating the excess as heat. Unlike with your car, however, when it comes to your metabolism, inefficiency is a *good* thing. It will coax your body into burning more calories—and more fat—for fuel.

- **Boost the number of calories your body burns through movement.** Thanks to that desk job, family commitments, and great lineup of must-see TV, most of us move less at ages 30, 40, and beyond than we did during our teens and twenties. The Metabolism Advantage plan reverses that trend, challenging you to exercise at least 5 hours each week. (As I've already mentioned, this should increase calorie burning by about 300 to 600 calories per day).

All told, you can expect to increase your daily calorie burn by between 40 and 60 percent within just 8 weeks. In other words, a guy who currently burns 2,500 calories a day would rev up his metabolism to a 3,400 to 4,000 daily calorie burn! That's enough of a boost for you to see a 10-to-15-pound drop in body fat if you work hard at it. Even more important, the Metabolism Advantage plan will simultaneously help you improve your health. In addition to speeding your metabolism, building muscle, and shedding fat, you can also expect to lower your blood cholesterol, blood pressure, and blood sugar. You can expect to not only look better but also live longer.

So, in the end, large-scale metabolic decline isn't inevitable. If you fight a good fight against metabolic slowdown, you can win the war. *The Metabolism Advantage* provides you with the fail-proof battle plan to make that happen. Throughout the pages of this book, you'll find everything you need to know about eating, exercising, and supplementing to maintain the metabolism of your twenties.

What are you waiting for? Isn't it about time you turned back the clock on your metabolism?

1

Metabolism for Life

An inside look at how your body burns calories

Remember when you were 20 years young and could eat pretty much anything you wanted? Back then, you didn't have to worry about going to the gym regularly or watching what you ate. You looked in the mirror and saw a great body—every day. The best part? It just seemed to come naturally.

Within a few years, though, things started to change, didn't they? Now, in your late twenties, thirties, forties, or beyond, you look in the mirror and wonder where that body went. Perhaps you need a new mirror.

Or perhaps you need a new approach.

Before you can understand how to reverse this age-related trend, you must first understand what your metabolism is and how it works. When it comes to these matters, I've determined that most people are pretty fuzzy—at best. Where is the metabolism? Is it stationed somewhere in your head, heart, or stomach? What does your metabolism do? Does it burn calories, fat, or protein?

Indeed, when most people think of metabolism, they think of the body's ability to burn calories or fat. Unfortunately, this definition is as limited as thinking of New York City as the place where the Statue of Liberty lifts her torch. Of course, New York City is home to the Statue of Liberty, and your metabolism does help you burn fat and calories, but both have so much more to offer.

You will be able to understand how to use the Metabolism Advantage only once you understand how your metabolism works. So, with no further ado, let's get started on this biology 101 lesson. I promise I'll keep things simple. Read and learn. What you discover in the following pages will help increase your success in your quest.

What Is Metabolism?

Scientists define metabolism as the chemical processes inside living cells that are necessary for the maintenance of life. Because you have living cells in your skin, blood, brain, and internal organs, your metabolism is literally ever present throughout your body. It's not in your brain, heart, or stomach. It's in your cells, all 100 trillion of them.

Inside each and every cell in your body are small structures called mitochondria, and they represent your main metabolic machinery. They are the powerhouses of your body, turning the calories that you eat into energy. That's why many people think of calorie burning when they hear the word *metabolism*. The mitochondria literally take food and burn it up to produce energy.

SCIENCE MADE SIMPLE

METABOLISM: The chemical processes inside living cells that are necessary for the maintenance of life

---

These tiny structures do much more than simply burn calories, however. They break down some compounds (proteins, carbohydrates, and fats) to yield energy for vital processes, and they build

THE STORY OF THE HUMBLE CARROT

To give you a specific example of how your metabolism keeps you alive and gives you energy, let's take a look at what might happen to a carrot after you chew it up and swallow.

The carrot is simple, fibrous, and quite nutritious, loaded with energy, vitamins, and minerals. Although it has some good stuff in it, that stuff isn't usable by your body until after the processes of digestion and metabolism occur. Therefore, you chew the carrot and swallow, and it enters the stomach, where acids break down the starchy carbohydrates into simple sugars, vitamins, and minerals. This whole process is necessary so that the sugars, vitamins, and minerals can travel—through the blood—to the cells, where they can be of real benefit.

Once the digested carrot chemicals hit your cells, the sugars can have one of several fates.

First, if you're active and your body requires energy to perform movement or rebuild itself from prior exercise, the sugar undergoes a metabolic process called catabolism. Catabolism is breaking down, and in this case, the sugar is broken down to release energy. Since the chemical bonds in sugar contain lots of energy, metabolizing sugar gives you a lot of energy if it's needed.

This sugar can have two other fates, one very undesirable. If you're not active and your body doesn't need any more energy than it already has, this sugar will most likely be metabolized through a process known as anabolism. Anabolism is building up, and in this case, the sugar is built up into a more complex carbohydrate and stored as glycogen in the liver or muscle. Alternatively—and you're not going to like this—it can be stored (after another metabolic process) in fat cells.

What about the other nutrients in carrots, such as vitamin A? Surprise—carrots don't actually contain vitamin A. Instead, they contain a natural chemical called beta-carotene, also called pro-vitamin A. After digestion, the beta-carotene travels to the cells, where it can be metabolized into vitamin A, a nutrient important for night vision, healthy skin, immune function, antioxidant protection, and much more.

Now you can see why metabolism is so important. It takes chemicals that your body can't necessarily use and helps convert them to chemicals that it can use. When metabolism functions optimally, you have better repair, more energy, and, of course, the ability to outwit Elmer Fudd.

other compounds to form substances essential to life (hormones like testosterone and estrogen). So, as you might imagine (and you're doing so because your brain is now metabolizing energy, producing thought), your mitochondria are very important structures.

Now, when you're young, your mitochondria tend to work well, making energy, burning calories, and keeping you lean and healthy. As you age, however, nasty free radicals proliferate. These unstable molecules are missing an electron. When a free radical forms, it tries to replace its missing electron and regain stability by attacking the nearest stable molecule and stealing one of its electrons. The attacked molecule then becomes a free radical itself, and a destructive cycle begins. In their search for electrons, free radicals often damage healthy molecules—including your mitochondria. More specifically, free radicals bombard the genetic material (DNA) contained within your mitochondria. In doing so, they alter your youthful response to calorie intake.

With somewhere between 10 trillion and 100 trillion cells in your body, you've got a lot of mitochondria and a lot of calorie-burning power. If you don't take care of these metabolic powerhouses, however, they will dwindle in number and capacity, reducing your overall metabolism. The Metabolism Advantage plan, among other things, helps preserve your mitochondria. It both feeds them the nutrition they need to fend off free radical attacks and exercises them (since, as with the rest of your body, if you don't use them, you'll lose them).

The Four Components of Metabolism

Simply put, your metabolism encompasses all of the breakdown and buildup reactions in your body. Now, I know you're mainly interested in one aspect of your metabolism: calorie burning. You picked up this book because you want to burn more calories and, as a result, burn off your blubber.

So let's talk about calories. Your metabolic rate is made up of the calories it takes to keep you alive, the calories you burn while exercising, the calories you burn while eating, and a small number of calories you burn based on your genetic makeup. Let's take a closer look at each.

1. TO KEEP YOU ALIVE

In scientific circles, this is known as your *resting metabolic rate (RMR)*. RMR represents the amount of energy it takes to do all the little physiological housekeeping chores inside your body, such as pumping blood, repairing tissues, and thinking. Your resting metabolism includes only those calories you burn at rest. It doesn't include the calories your muscles burn to power movement. (That's your physical activity level, or PAL.)

RMR represents the bulk (about 60 to 75 percent) of your total daily calorie burning. Because RMR is a major portion of your total metabolism, you're going to focus a lot of your energy on increasing it.

SCIENCE MADE SIMPLE

RESTING METABOLIC RATE (RMR): The amount of energy your body uses for basic operating functions, such as pumping blood, repairing tissues, and thinking

---

2. DURING EXERCISE AND MOVEMENT

Every time your muscles contract to power a movement—whether lifting and lowering your fingers during typing or moving your legs back and forth during walking—they burn calories. Your *physical activity level (PAL)* makes up between 15 and 30 percent of your total daily calorie burning, depending on whether or not you exercise. Of course, PAL doesn't include just going to the gym and exercising. It takes into account any movement at all, from standing and walking slowly to purposeful exercise. The Metabolism Advantage plan includes up to six workouts a week so you can make the most of this PAL burn.

SCIENCE MADE SIMPLE

PHYSICAL ACTIVITY LEVEL (PAL): The calories your body burns during exercise and other movement

---

3. WHILE EATING

You burn calories as you chew, swallow, and digest your food, a component of the metabolism known as the *thermic effect of feeding (TEF)*. After meals, your metabolism speeds up as your stomach churns, your digestive juices flow, and the tiny muscles along the lining of your intestines push food downstream. Your metabolism also speeds up due to the processing of the food: From the storage of some calories to the burning of others, anytime you eat, you burn some calories. This is why you may feel hot after eating a big meal.

SCIENCE MADE SIMPLE

THERMIC EFFECT OF FEEDING (TEF): The calories you burn to chew, swallow, and digest your food

---

TEF represents 5 to 15 percent of your total daily calorie burning, depending on how often and what you eat. Eat the right foods at the right times, and you can maximize your TEF, boosting total metabolism. The Metabolism Advantage plan maximizes your intake of the right foods and teaches you the right times to eat them—such as eating high-protein foods at every meal to boost TEF to the max.

4. GENETIC MAKEUP

Nonexercise activity thermogenesis (NEAT) represents approximately 5 percent of total daily calorie burning and is highly variable based on your genetic makeup. This one is pretty hard to change, so you won't focus much of your energy here.

The Reason You Burn Fat

Now you understand how and why your metabolism burns calories. Your body can burn calories from any of the three macronutrients: protein, fat, and carbohydrate. You want, of course, to burn more and more fat calories, especially those stored on your hips, thighs, and stomach. So now it's time for an important lesson—perhaps the most important lesson of this entire book. Remember this one:

> YOUR BODY IS NOT WASTEFUL.
> IT WILL BURN FAT ONLY WHEN IT NEEDS ENERGY.

In other words, you can't burn fat without increasing your body's need for energy. The bonds in carbohydrates and fats contain stored energy waiting to be used. Your body, however, will break these bonds and liberate this energy only if it really needs it. Doing the opposite—liberating all this energy when it doesn't need it—is just foolish. It would be the equivalent of running your heater on high with the windows open at noon on a hot summer day. You don't need the heat!

Want to know how to lose weight easily and effectively? Simply create a high energy need in your body. Do this, and you won't have to struggle to lose weight. Your metabolism will anxiously, even greedily, gobble up body fat, leaving you with a lean physique. Sounds appealing, right?

So how do you create an energy need? Well, here are some times when your body's needs for energy (and your metabolism) are high.

During exercise: Depending on the type of exercise, you can increase your body's energy requirement by 2-to-20-fold. That's a lot of calorie burning! Remember, though, you're not exercising all day. In fact, you'll probably exercise for only 1 hour or less each day. What about the other 23 hours? I'll talk about those in a second.

After exercise: During the first hour or two after intense exercise (interval exercise and weight lifting), your body's energy requirement remains high. This is called the afterburn effect. The afterburn, while highest within the first 1 to 2 hours after exercise, can persist for up to 24 hours. Add this extra calorie burn to the exercise calorie-burning effect, and you'll lose body fat—fast.

During repair: When you damage your body (for better or worse), your energy needs increase dramatically. Get the flu, and your body needs lots of energy. Break your leg, and your body needs lots of energy. Of course, these are not preferred methods of weight loss. Instead of asking your friends to sneeze on you in the name of weight loss, you can just head to your local gym. When you challenge your muscles to lift weights that are heavier than they are accustomed to lifting, your body undergoes small amounts of healthy muscle damage. This damage is costly to repair, and as a result, you get a great boost in metabolism. Because it can take as long as 7 days for your body to completely repair your muscles after an intense weightlifting session, this repair process creates a metabolism boost that lasts 24 hours a day, 7 days a week.

When eating "costly" foods: Some foods actually cost a lot—in terms of energy—to digest and metabolize. Proteins are a great example. Your body burns twice as many calories to digest high-protein foods as it does for high-carbohydrate or high-fat foods. This extra calorie burning adds up over time. Eat more energy-costly foods on a regular basis, and you'll rev up your metabolism on a regular basis.

When you have more muscle: All organs in your body regularly perform routine remodeling and upkeep on their cells. This daily demolition and building process burns calories. Your muscles are no exception: They burn a great number of calories to maintain themselves, regularly breaking down and building up new proteins. As a result, 1 extra pound of muscle may burn up to 50 extra calories—even while you're just sitting around watching TV.

Your Age and Your Metabolism

If you're in your thirties, forties, fifties, or beyond, it should come as no surprise that *something* happened as you got older. Even though you ate the same foods and exercised the same amount as you did during your twenties, you slowly grew larger with each passing year. One

WHERE, OH, WHERE DID YOUR METABOLISM GO?

As you age, if you don't take any steps, your metabolic rate takes a nose-dive. In fact, from the age of 25 until the age of 65, most people experience a slow, progressive loss of metabolic power. Without a plan, by the time you're 65, you'll be burning roughly 500 fewer calories daily than you did at 25. This reduction comes predominantly from a loss of RMR, but reductions in PAL, TEF, and NEAT also play a role, as the graph below shows.

Here's the good news: You don't have to resign yourself to this loss of metabolic power. It's not inevitable. By using the nutrition, exercise, and supplementation strategies in this book, you can match or even exceed the metabolism of your younger days.

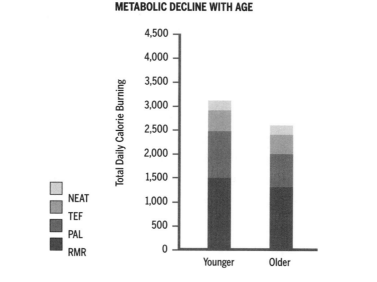

METABOLIC DECLINE WITH AGE

day, you looked in the mirror and wondered whose belly, whose hips, whose thighs were staring back at you. Then you bought this book. . . .

Or something like that.

But I digress. The point is, even though you seemingly were doing all the right things, your metabolism still slowed down. What happened? You didn't start eating more. You didn't start exercising less. So why did you gain so much weight?

Well, research has demonstrated that as you get older, the following things tend to occur.

You become less active. As you get older, you simply get too busy with work, family, and other responsibilities, and you don't make as much time for physical activity. Even if you still manage to do formal exercise for the same amount of time as when you were younger, overall you're probably less active during the course of the day. For example, when you have a desk job, you walk around much less often than you did during high school or college, when you used the shoe leather express to get from one class to another.

You eat fewer calories and eat at the wrong times. Although you might think that eating less would help prevent weight gain, it actually slows your metabolism. Our not-so-distant pre-industrial ancestors survived by hunting and gathering and consequently feasted and starved on a regular basis. Those whose bodies lowered their metabolisms during famine tended to survive and pass on their genes. As a result, modern-day humans have a quite sensitive mechanism that fairly quickly turns down metabolism when it senses that fewer calories are coming in. When you go too many hours without eating or dramatically reduce your overall calorie intake, your brain tells the cells in your body to slow down the works, and you burn fewer overall calories as a result. Your body also starts to burn carbohydrates and muscle protein for energy, preserving your fat. Less muscle equals a permanently lowered RMR.

Restricting calories slows metabolism for yet another, lesser known reason: It reduces your overall metabolic flux. Metabolic flux? If you're not familiar with this concept, don't worry. Most people, including many of the scientists, exercise specialists, and nutritionists I regularly encounter, haven't heard of it either. Despite its relative obscurity *today*, this concept will have a big impact on how people develop their health and body composition strategies in the future. So, in a few years, when your friends start gushing about metabolic flux and how you can boost it to trigger weight loss, you can sit back confidently and say, "Oh, that? I've known about *that* for ages."

The definition of *flux* is "flow," so metabolic flux is the same thing as metabolic flow, or the flow of energy into and out of your body. Energy flows into the metabolic systems of your body when you eat, and it flows out of them when you burn calories (through planned exercise and daily movement). It's this relationship between flux in and flux out that equals metabolic flux.

When you put more energy into the system (by eating more) and take more energy out of the system (by exercising more), you increase your flux. Consequently, your metabolism must work harder to process all of those calories. The higher your flux, the higher your metabolism.

An interesting study published in 2004 determined the following: When you take someone who has a high metabolic flux and slow down that flux, you can do the opposite of what we're trying to do— you can actually turn down your metabolism!

In this study, researchers asked 10 men who were in energy balance at about 2,300 calories per day (meaning their intake and expenditure were both in the 2,300 range) to reduce their metabolic flux. To accomplish this, the men restricted both their food intake and exercise expenditure, achieving a new energy balance of 1,800 calories per day. Consequently, their metabolic rates dropped, meaning that even in energy balance, the body prefers a higher metabolic flux.

The authors of this study wrote, "High energy flux is a key mech-

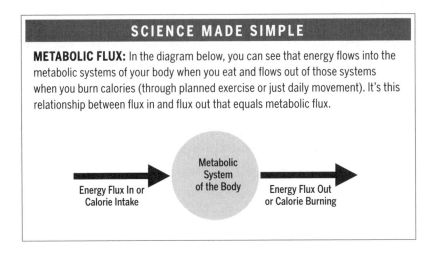
anism contributing to the elevated RMR . . . in habitually exercising older adults. Maintenance of high energy flux via regular exercise may be an effective strategy for maintaining energy expenditure and preventing age-associated obesity."

As you can see, eating (and exercising) less acts as a big ingredient in the recipe for a sluggish metabolism and a bunch of weight gain.

You lose lean body mass. With less activity, more stress, and fewer calories, you can say bye-bye to the firm body of your youth. Even if you weren't muscle-bound as a young person, you did have more muscle than you do now.

The human body is programmed to build and maintain muscle during the early adult years. From there, unless you take steps to prevent it, your body drops lean body mass (muscle, bone, and other nonfat tissue) at a rate of about 5 to 10 pounds every 10 years. According to research, adults lose, on average, 25 pounds of lean body mass between ages 25 and 65.

Muscle loss doesn't just add up to a poor placing at the Mr. Universe contest. It also means last place in the Mr. Metabolism contest. Scientists have estimated that the RMR (the part of your metabolism that accounts for about 60 to 75 percent of all the calories you burn each day) is highly dependent on muscle mass. In fact, 75 to 80 percent of your RMR is determined by your muscle mass. The more muscle you have, the higher the RMR. The less muscle you have, the lower the RMR.

So what happens when you become less active, eat less, eat at the wrong times, and lose muscle? Do I really have to tell you? Take a look in the mirror and see for yourself.

That's right, you gain weight, body parts start to sag, your health starts to decline, and you have a lot less energy than when you were younger. The average person who becomes less active, eats differently, and loses muscle experiences a 20 to 25 percent drop in 24-hour metabolism (measured as 24-hour energy expenditure) at some point between the ages of 25 and 65. This adds up to a daily metabolic decrease of more than 500 calories a day.

Now, if you don't know the body composition impact of 500 calories, check out these scary numbers.

500 calories per day x 7 days per week = 3,500 calories per week
3,500 calories = 1 pound of fat

That's right, according to these calculations, if you let your metabolism decline to this level, you can expect to gain in the neighborhood of 1 pound of fat per week *while* losing muscle. No wonder people look worse as they age.

Rev Up Your Health

With all this discussion of body composition, fat burning, and muscle, you might think the Metabolism Advantage plan is only about vanity, about looking better naked. That couldn't be further from the truth. Yes, you *will* look better naked, partially dressed, and fully dressed. Your friends, family, and co-workers will notice how fantastic you look, and you'll feel stronger than you ever have before. Your metabolism, however, is about much more than how you look. It's about your health and about how you live.

The Metabolism Advantage plan is about adding years to your life, adding life to your years, improving your ability to do the everyday tasks you want to do whenever you want to do them, staying out of the doctor's office, getting off your medications, and living the life you want to live without worrying about your body stopping short.

For example, one of my clients, Daniel, started his Metabolism Advantage program at age 32. At this young age, he had already had two heart attacks and was struggling to get his cholesterol levels down through exercise and diet. "I tried statins [cholesterol-lowering drugs] but found that I couldn't tolerate the side effects," he told me. "I started following your exercise and nutrition plan religiously and, even though I wasn't fat, lost 10 pounds of bad weight during the first month and cut my LDL cholesterol in half over 6 months! My doctors are amazed that I could make this type of improvement with diet and exercise and are now advising me against other drug therapies."

He's just one of many clients who revved up not only their metabolisms but also their health. Diabetes, cardiovascular disease, and obesity are all diseases of metabolism. A sluggish, dysfunctional metabolism raises your risk for all three, a deadly condition known as syndrome X. Fix your metabolism with the Metabolism Advantage plan, and you may prevent—and even treat—these metabolic disorders.

Let's take a closer look at just one of these diseases, diabetes. Although many people think diabetes is one of those diseases your grandma gets, very few realize just how prevalent this metabolically and physically destructive disease is. First of all, type 2 diabetes affects approximately 18.2 million people, or 6.3 percent of the population, in the United States. That's either an impossible number of grandmas or just a big portion of non-grandma population. Type 2 diabetes used to be called adult-onset diabetes because at one time, it

THE METABOLISM ADVANTAGE PROMISE

Lots of programs claim to improve the way your body looks (body composition), but many of these programs don't necessarily impact the way your body feels (health) or moves (physical performance). In the diagram below, these programs fall into Zone A. Want to hear the scary part? Some of the programs in Zone A can actually degrade health and physical performance. That's quite a price to pay for looking better!

Of course, there are many other programs designed to improve your overall health. Unfortunately, many of those won't really impact the way your body looks or the way it moves. In the diagram below, these programs fall into Zone B.

Finally, there are programs out there that are supposed to improve physical performance without necessarily improving health or body composition. In the diagram below, these programs fall into Zone C.

Frustrating, isn't it? Well, you don't have to be frustrated any longer. The Metabolism Advantage plan helps you to reach the *intersection* of these three goals. Now you can achieve optimal body composition, optimal health, and optimal physical performance. The Metabolism Advantage falls into Zone D, and this zone is so small because so few programs out there actually cut it. Want to achieve this perfect intersection? Keep turning the pages.

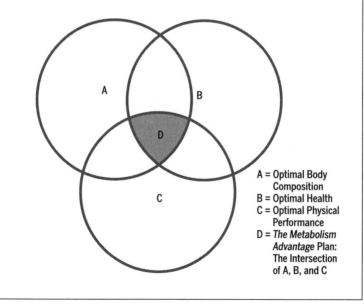

A = Optimal Body
    Composition
B = Optimal Health
C = Optimal Physical
    Performance
D = *The Metabolism
    Advantage* Plan:
    The Intersection
    of A, B, and C

didn't affect people until after the age of 45. Today, more and more younger people are being diagnosed with it. At least 2 percent of the 20-to-39-year-old crowd has type 2 diabetes, with more than 200,000 new cases diagnosed each year. Pediatricians have diagnosed the disease in children as young as age 4! It's a true epidemic, and something people of all ages should take steps to prevent.

If you're overweight, even if you "just have a few pounds to lose," you're at risk of developing this awful condition. Although you may not technically have diabetes—yet—you may have chronically high insulin levels or other metabolic problems that increase your risk of developing diabetes down the road.

Since you're reading this book, I'm going to take a wild guess and assume that you've got a few pounds to lose. Read the following paragraphs closely, because in addition to revving up your metabolism, you also need to reduce your risk of diabetes.

Diabetes is the sixth most common cause of death in the United States. And doctors are only now realizing that many of the deaths they see and attribute to other causes are really diabetes related. Some of the problems associated with diabetes include:

- Heart disease and stroke
- High blood pressure
- Blindness
- Kidney disease
- Nervous system disease
- Amputations
- Dental disease
- Pregnancy complications

The Metabolism Advantage plan will help you prevent diabetes by improving the effectiveness of the hormone insulin inside your body. When you eat, the amount of carbohydrate (sugar) in your blood rises, even if you haven't actually eaten sugar. In response, your pancreas secretes insulin, a hormone that escorts sugar into hungry

Since I'm a visual learner, I always enjoy looking at diagrams and pictures. If you're like me, you'll appreciate the graph below. It shows how the four components of metabolism add up in sedentary and physically active people. Note that nearly all components of metabolism are higher in the active group as compared with the sedentary group. Consequently, the active individuals burn more total calories in a day. When you're active, your PAL goes up, and so do your RMR, your TEF, and your NEAT. Now that is neat!

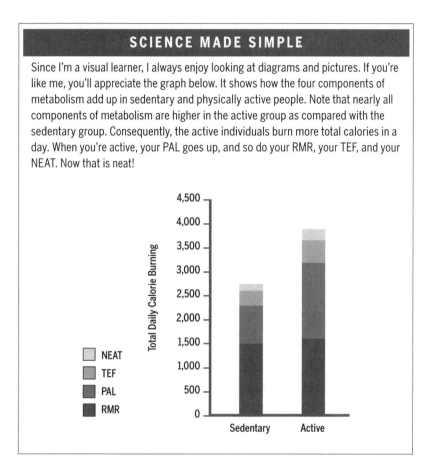

cells that either burn it for energy or store it for later use. Insulin can escort sugar to any number of places, ranging from your liver and muscles to other bodily cells, including fat cells.

The Metabolism Advantage exercise plan will condition your muscle cells to respond to insulin more quickly so that they more easily open their doors and let sugar in to be burned for energy. This increased insulin sensitivity reduces the amount of insulin that your pancreas must secrete to clear blood sugar. The end result: Insulin and blood sugar levels go down.

Type 2 diabetes is a preventable, modifiable, and even reversible condition. The strategies laid out in this book will help you prevent and/or treat diabetes. You see, research has demonstrated that you must do the following to prevent this disease.

- Exercise for 30 to 60 minutes daily
- Strength train at least 2 days a week
- Lose weight (yep, weight loss is a treatment for diabetes)
- Increase protein intake to knock some carbohydrates out of your diet
- Increase consumption of high-fiber foods to eliminate some sugary foods from your diet

The same prescription outlined above also boosts metabolism. All of the strategies in this book that improve metabolism have also been shown to reduce diabetes risk and/or diabetes symptoms. So you'll not only boost that waning metabolic rate but also kick diabetes to the curb.

2

The Metabolism Advantage Formula

A three-pronged approach to rebuilding the metabolism of your twenties

Now that you understand all of the ways in which your body burns calories, it's time for you to find out how to coax those various calorie-burning systems into burning *even more*.

I'm not going to sugarcoat things for you. The Metabolism Advantage plan requires time, determination, and sweat. You must eat the right foods at the right times, work out for 5 hours a week, and take a few supplements religiously. Yet the hard work you put into this program will pay off in huge rewards. Within the next 8 weeks, you are going to speed up your metabolism by about 50 percent, totaling between 1,000 and 1,500 calories a day. That's enough to incinerate 1 to 2 pounds of fat from your frame each week. Most exciting? You'll be eating *more* as you do it. You'll shed fat and build muscle *without hunger*.

The Metabolism Advantage plan is based on a three-part equation that adds up to a faster metabolism. It works like this:

Metabolism Advantage eating + Metabolism Advantage supplements + Metabolism Advantage exercise = The metabolism of your twenties

The three elements of the equation work together symbiotically. Your nutrition plan and supplement plan support your exercise plan, and vice versa. Think of eating, supplementing, and exercising as a three-legged stool. The seat of the stool—your metabolism—needs all three legs for support. Remove any of the legs, and the stool topples.

Let's take a closer look at how each leg of the program adds up to a faster metabolism, starting with Metabolism Advantage nutrition.

Get the Advantage with Food

Over the years, you've probably responded to the extra fat growing around your middle in a perfectly understandable way. You ate less. You cut back on your beer drinking, halved your servings of fries, and possibly even skipped a meal from time to time. Although these methods may have helped you to temporarily shed fat, they put the brakes on your metabolism.

Indeed, you must eat *more* rather than *less*. On the Metabolism Advantage nutrition plan, you will eat every 2 to 3 hours, filling your plate with foods that support muscle growth, making your body a less efficient calorie burner, boosting metabolism, and increasing the calories you burn during the process of digestion.

Remember the concept of metabolic flux that I mentioned in Chapter 1? Just in case you don't, it works like this: Energy flows into the metabolic systems of your body when you eat and flows out of them when you burn calories (through planned exercise or just daily movement). When you put more energy into the system (by eating more) and take more out (by moving more), you increase your flux.

Consequently, your metabolism must work harder to process all of those calories. The higher your flux, the higher your metabolism.

The very nature of this increase in flux (more energy being added, more being broken down) boosts your metabolism, causing your cells to waste calories as heat. It also helps shift your body composition, stimulating your cells to burn through more fat and store more carbohydrates and protein. More food equals more metabolism. More exercise equals hungrier muscle tissue. The two translate to more fat burning and more muscle building. It all works together. In short, by increasing your flux, you feed your muscles and starve your fat.

As a side benefit, you also improve your health and may even extend your life. By eating more of the right types of food, you'll consume more health-promoting vitamins, minerals, and other nutrients. You'll also speed up the turnover of body tissues. By exercising and eating more (thereby increasing your flux), you break down the tissues you have today and create new, better-adapted ones for tomorrow. This leads to a constantly rejuvenated body, one that will last longer and perform better.

On the Metabolism Advantage plan, you'll probably eat more food more often than you do now. As a result, you'll speed up your metabolism, shed fat, and build muscle—*without being hungry*.

In addition to eating more food, you'll also eat *better* food. Each week, you'll eat several servings of Metabolism Advantage Metafoods such as lean red meat, spinach, and avocado. You'll build your meals around muscle-stimulating lean protein and metabolism-boosting veggies. In this way, you'll provide your muscles with the fuel they need to grow, supporting your efforts in the gym.

Many people think of weightlifting when they think of muscle building, but that's only one piece of the muscle-building puzzle. Building muscle in the absence of the right nutrition program is about as easy as getting tickets to the opening ceremonies at the Olympics. In order to supercharge your strength-training workouts, the Metabolism Advantage nutrition plan incorporates the following three nutritional essentials.

1. ADEQUATE TOTAL ENERGY INTAKE

Studies at Tufts University show that the calories required for weight maintenance increase by 15 percent on a strengthening program. To build muscle, you'll need even more calories. That said, pigging out on 20 percent more dinner isn't the way to get those calories. The additional energy intake must be dispersed throughout the day and must come from the right foods.

2. ADEQUATE PROTEIN INTAKE

Muscles are made up of protein, and studies done at Purdue University show that the Recommended Dietary Allowance (RDA) for protein simply isn't enough to prevent age-related muscle loss. This is why the Metabolism Advantage plan recommends eating protein with every meal and/or snack and that some of this protein come from animal sources (like meat, chicken, fish, eggs, and dairy foods). In studies completed at the University of Arkansas for Medical Sciences, participants who ate a varied diet that contained meat increased lean body mass and lost body fat during 12 weeks of strengthening exercise. On the other hand, participants who ate a varied diet containing the same amount of protein but no meat actually lost lean body mass.

3. ADEQUATE MICRONUTRIENT INTAKE

Typically, vitamin and mineral intake varies with total calorie intake. Assuming you make good food choices, as calorie intake goes up, vitamin and mineral intake also goes up. As calorie intake goes down, so does vitamin and mineral intake. This becomes an important relationship as we age. With each passing decade, both men and women tend to eat less. This lower-calorie diet results in getting fewer micronutrients (vitamins and minerals).

Why should you care about vitamins and minerals? Well, while micronutrients don't provide energy or build muscle directly, they do *support* the production of energy, the building of muscle, and the maintenance of health. Vitamins and minerals play these key roles because they are co-factors in many of the chemical and metabolic reactions in the body, making them necessary for optimal metabolic function.

Unfortunately, when older people combine lower energy intake with poor food choices, they can end up very undernourished from a micronutrient perspective. According to research done at Purdue, as we age, we need to be more conscious of our intakes of the following micronutrients: vitamins B_2 (riboflavin), B_6, B_{12}, D, and E; the B vitamin folate; and the minerals calcium and iron. The Metabolism Advantage food plan maximizes these nutrients.

Get the Advantage with Supplements

In recent years, the supplement industry has taken a beating from the government and the media. If you've been following the news, you've probably read the many accounts about supplements that don't work, supplements that are dangerous, supplements that contain impurities, and supplements that don't contain the ingredients they advertise.

Such reports have cast a dark cloud over all supplements. This is too bad because some supplements have downright amazing effects on metabolism. On the Metabolism Advantage plan, you'll use five supplements religiously.

1. Fish oil
2. Protein supplements
3. Greens supplements
4. Creatine
5. Postworkout recovery drinks

Unlike the supplements you may have read about in the media, these are safe, effective, and good for you. They will harmonize with your nutrition and exercise plans to produce fast, healthy, impressive results.

When you use all five Metabolism Advantage supplements daily, you provide your body with important muscle-building and fat-burning nutrients that are nearly impossible to get from food alone. The supplements boost metabolism, stimulate fat burning, and set the stage for muscle growth. They also provide wonderful side effects such as better blood sugar control, reduced blood cholesterol levels, increased energy, stronger bones, and improved memory. Simply put, these nutrients have repeatedly been shown to offer benefits in terms of health, body composition, and performance.

Get the Advantage with Exercise

The main Metabolism Advantage exercise plan includes three 45-minute-to-1-hour strength-training sessions and three 25-to-30-minute cardio sessions each week. This amount of exercise will burn 2,000 calories or more during your workouts each week.

That's *a lot* of calorie burning, for sure. But the Metabolism Advantage exercise plan gives you an additional calorie-burning edge.

These workouts will help you build back some of the lean mass (muscle, bone, and other nonfat tissues) that you've lost over the years. That's a critical ingredient in rediscovering the metabolism of your youth.

In Chapter 1, you learned that the average person can lose 25 pounds of lean mass between ages 25 and 65. With the right exercise, however, you can reverse this trend. According to research, people who—through exercise and smart eating—maintain their lean mass as they age experience only a 0.36 percent drop in metabolism per decade as compared with the usual 5 to 7 percent drop that most aging adults experience. So by exercising and preserving your muscle mass, you can save at least 10 times as much metabolic power as your nonexercising friends. If they lose 500 or more calories of metabolic

FRINGE BENEFITS OF A STRONGER BODY

Muscle building doesn't mean only bulking up, lifting cars, and stretching shirtsleeves. If you eat and exercise the right way, muscle building adds up to a lean body, a smaller waist, smaller clothing sizes, and the defiance of gravity. In fact, in addition to helping you to look better, weightlifting will do the following:

✓ Increase overall strength and ability to perform daily tasks
✓ Increase bone density and bone strength
✓ Reduce arthritis pain
✓ Increase glucose tolerance (blood sugar regulation)
✓ Reduce back pain
✓ Improve digestion

If you follow the Metabolism Advantage plan, building muscle through strengthening exercise won't make you bulky. Rather, it will jumpstart your metabolism and have you looking great in no time.

OF MUSCLE AND METABOLISM

In the graph below, you can see that as fat-free mass (muscle mass) increases, resting metabolic rate (RMR) also increases. When muscle mass decreases, so does RMR. Even if you're not a "graph person," the message is clear: The 25-pound loss in muscle mass that many people experience between the ages of 25 and 65 can lead to a 20 percent reduction in metabolic power.

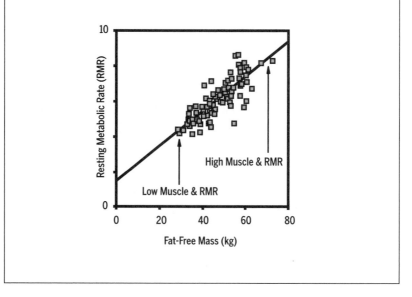

power from age 25 to 65, you'll lose only 50 calories. Want even better news? With the targeted approach the Metabolism Advantage plan offers, I'll teach you how to prevent even that 50-calorie loss. Follow the three-step Metabolism Advantage approach, and you can rev your metabolism to a rate that's even higher than what you had in your twenties!

The Metabolism Advantage exercise plan will help you build and maintain muscle through a series of targeted weight-training workouts designed to fully stimulate all of your muscle fibers. Contrary to popular opinion, weightlifting *is* for everyone—men and women, young and old, bodybuilders and computer programmers.

Most important, you're never too old to turn back the clock. As a PhD student at the University of Western Ontario, I was privy to a fantastic experiment at the Canadian Centre for Activity and Aging (CCAA) that arrived at this very conclusion. The CCAA in London, Ontario, offered extensive programs in strength training, cardiovascular conditioning, osteoporosis risk prevention, hip fracture rehabilitation, functional fitness, and stress management for seniors. At any given time, you could wander over to the CCAA to watch people of all ages—even some in their nineties—strength training their way to better, healthier, more functional bodies.

Now, although it may be hard to imagine a group of 70-, 80-, and 90-year-olds hefting weights, it can—and does—happen, and not just in Canada. In community programs around the world, seniors are finally recognizing the value of strength training and are performing some of the same lifting movements that linebackers and professional wrestlers do. And the results? The seniors in the CCAA and many other experiments reaped the following benefits.

- They gained 3 pounds of lean mass in 8 weeks. That's enough to counteract almost a decade's worth of neglect.
- They boosted resting metabolism by 7 percent and total metabolism by 15 percent. Since the average person loses about 5 to 7 percent of their metabolism per decade, this is enough to undo two decades of damage.
- They also shed fat, strengthened their bones, reduced their blood pressure, experienced less back pain, and found relief from painful conditions such as rheumatoid arthritis, osteoarthritis, and fibromyalgia.

With this list of benefits, what are you waiting for? Your grandma is strength training—why aren't you?

By now, I hope you're convinced that muscle is your friend. It not only keeps you looking and feeling good but also keeps you healthy and revs up your metabolism.

In addition to building muscle through strength training, you'll also boost your metabolism through intense cardiovascular workouts. The Metabolism Advantage cardio plan prescribes interval training. In these high-intensity workouts, you'll alternate between surges of fast-paced cardio and a slower recovery pace. Research shows that this type of intense cardio can rev up your metabolism not only during your workouts but also for many hours afterward, as your body repairs and replenishes muscle tissue. All told, the Metabolism Advantage exercise plan will boost your calorie-burning potential during your workouts, after your workouts, and all day long.

A Three-Pronged Attack on Flab

Metabolism Advantage eating, supplementing, and exercising will help you boost all of the different aspects of metabolism that you learned about in Chapter 1. By boosting your overall calorie intake, exercising more often, and increasing your muscle mass, you'll boost your resting metabolic rate (RMR). The increased activity you'll take part in on the Metabolism Advantage plan will also boost your physical activity level (PAL). As we get older, we typically do less planned exercise (what we think of as working out) and unplanned exercise (everyday activities that require movement). The Metabolism Advantage plan will reverse that trend. Finally, the nutrition and exercise programs will also boost the thermic effect of feeding (TEF). As we age, we typically experience a double reduction in TEF. First, we eat less and less. Decreasing food intake and meal frequency decreases TEF. Second, since physical activity is linked to TEF, as our PAL drops, our TEF also drops. The Metabolism Advantage will turn that around as well. All told, you'll be incinerating calories like never before.

You'll tackle the plan in two phases. Phase 1 spans 8 weeks, during which you'll follow a specific meal plan and workout schedule

THE NUMBERS GAME

The Metabolism Advantage is a book filled with estimates and numbers. For example, I estimate that you'll boost your overall metabolism by 40 to 60 percent in 8 weeks. I estimate that, after 8 weeks, your body will burn 1,000 to 1,500 more calories a day. You'll read about a study that found that fish oil boosts metabolism by roughly 400 calories daily. You'll find out roughly how many calories you'll burn during your Metabolism Advantage workouts—as well as afterward. You'll find out how much lean body mass you can expect to build on the Metabolism Advantage plan, along with how many daily calories that lean mass will burn.

I have two points to make regarding these matters. First, resist the urge to add up and quantify all of the numbers. Various parts of the metabolism overlap, so just because studies have shown that fish oil boosts metabolism by 400 calories a day and just because you'll burn 300 or more calories during your Metabolism Advantage workouts, that doesn't mean you can add the two numbers together and come up with a daily metabolism boost of 700 calories. It just doesn't work that way.

Second, keep in mind that all of the numbers throughout this book are estimates. Each human body runs a little differently. Some people burn more calories; others burn fewer. Will you definitely burn 1,000 to 1,500 more calories a day by the end of this plan? It's likely, but maybe not. It really depends on a few things, such as how hard you work, the consistency of your efforts, and your individual genetics. I can, however, promise you this: If you follow the Metabolism Advantage program at least 90 percent of the time, you will speed up your metabolism in a big way. You will lose fat and build muscle, and you'll look better as a result. Numbers aside, isn't that all that matters?

designed to get you used to the Metabolism Advantage lifestyle in the most effortless way possible. You can either stick to the specific day-by-day blueprint that I've provided in Chapter 7, or you may modify the plan somewhat, using the advice from Chapter 9 to guide you. During phase 2—8 weeks and beyond—you'll maintain the healthful habits you formed during the previous weeks. When you tackle the plan in these two steps, you prevent the yo-yo effect. In phase 1, you *go on* the plan, then, in phase 2, you *stay on* the plan. Although phase 2 certainly provides more flexibility than phase 1, it doesn't allow for backsliding. To maintain your results, you must maintain the Metabolism Advantage lifestyle.

In the chapters that follow, you'll learn all the details you need for life. Whether you're 30, 40, 50, or beyond, you can turn back the clock on your metabolism. *The Metabolism Advantage* will show you how.

PART 2

THE TRINITY OF A GREAT METABOLISM

$$\boxed{3}$$

The Metabolism Advantage Nutrition Plan

The foods you need to feed your muscle and starve your fat

It should come as no surprise that to boost your metabolism and improve your health, body composition, and physical performance, you must watch what you eat. Unfortunately, "watching what you eat" has become synonymous with deprivation, tedium, and monotony.

In the name of weight loss, numerous diet plans have succeeded in turning a very simple process into a complicated mathematical equation requiring you to add up calories, "points," or grams of fat and carbohydrate—and sometimes all of these. They require you to measure precise amounts of food for every meal and painstakingly balance hard-to-define percentages of carbohydrates, proteins, and fats. Most disheartening: You must rid your kitchen of all sorts of so-called fattening foods.

By focusing on what you shouldn't eat (carbs, fats, foods worth too many points, or whatever), many diets cause you to think and dream about only one thing: your nutritional enemies. Don't let these diets scare you away from good nutrition. Eating for a faster metabolism and a leaner body need not be so complicated, time consuming, and downright distasteful.

The Metabolism Advantage provides a very different approach. You see, instead of subtraction, the Metabolism Advantage plan uses addition. Instead of giving up bad foods, you add good foods. Through a combination of displacement and timing, you'll consume the right foods at the right times to rev up your metabolism and ratchet down your appetite.

By focusing on eating *more* metabolism-boosting foods and not on eating *less* of other foods, you'll automatically eat fewer of the foods that contribute to fat gain, muscle loss, and a sluggish metabolism. Before we get into exactly how this works, however, let's first take a closer look at why cutting the bad foods from your diet doesn't work.

Why Dieting Makes You Fat

When most people think of the word *diet*, they think of deprivation, restrictions, and, ultimately, failure. Although technically, *diet* refers to a way of eating, it has colloquially come to define a *temporary* way of eating. You go on a diet. You lose weight. You go off the diet. You gain weight. You go on a diet. You lose weight. You go off the diet. You gain weight. The cycle continues.

Indeed, 90 percent of the people who lose weight on diets gain back some portion of it, and 30 percent regain more than they lost. For the following four reasons, dieting is the exact opposite of what you should be doing.

DIETING DECREASES YOUR METABOLISM

When you diet, you eat less. When you eat less, your metabolism slows. Why? First, when you eat less, you lower that all-important flux that I mentioned in chapters 1 and 2. You put less fuel into your metabolism, and as a result, you have less fuel to burn. Second, when you eat less, you reduce the thermic effect of feeding (TEF). Your body burns calories as you chew, swallow, and digest food, so when you eat less, you burn less—plain and simple. Finally, when you diet, your body starts to prepare for starvation, turning down the heat on your metabolism and encouraging your body to conserve calories. Your resting metabolic rate (RMR) and TEF are directly related to how much you eat, so if you eat less, RMR and TEF go down. Reduce these two large components of metabolism, and your ability to burn fat diminishes.

DIETING DECREASES YOUR MUSCLE MASS

Food powers your workouts. In order to have the energy to work out hard and the calories to build muscle, you need to eat enough food. When you lose weight through dieting, your body actually does everything it can to conserve your fat stores, so instead of burning fat, you burn muscle. Yes, you lose weight according to the scale, but you lose the wrong type of weight!

DIETS ARE TEMPORARY

For most people, dieting is a means to an end: weight loss. They think that once they reach their goals, they can just go back to eating as they did before. It doesn't work that way. If you "go on a diet" to lose weight, you'll undoubtedly drop some pounds. But, as the statistics I've already mentioned demonstrate, as soon as you go off the diet, you'll undoubtedly gain it back—which brings me to my final point.

DIETING = WEIGHT REGAIN

With a reduction in muscle and a reduction in metabolism, as soon as you stop dieting, you gain back the weight. Let's look at the fictional but typical tale of one dieter we'll call Mark. He's 5'11" and weighs 190 pounds. He'd like to get down to 170, his high school weight, so he begins to eat less. He cuts out a meal here and there. He avoids desserts. He skips dinner parties. He eats appetizers and salads instead of entrées. The weight slowly comes off, and the external changes make him happy.

If Mark could peek inside his body and see all the ramifications of his diet, however, he wouldn't be so happy. For starters, his brain is actually beginning to starve, making him feel less mentally sharp. In order to subtly encourage him to eat more, his brain begins to release hormones that increase appetite. Mark gets progressively hungrier and starts to feel daily cravings. Because his willpower is strong, though, he ignores them until he hits his "goal weight."

While he was losing weight, he didn't seem to be getting firmer. It's as if he's become just a smaller version of his previously "soft" self. He can wear those old jeans from high school, but they just don't fit the same. Although he is down to the same weight he was in high school, he looks different—softer.

What happened? Well, Mark's body began to break down muscle for energy. If he had been exercising properly, his body would have spared that muscle. He hasn't been challenging those muscles to work every day, however, so his body decided that having all that muscle was a waste of energy. As I've mentioned, muscle is the body's main metabolic machinery, accounting for more than 60 percent of total daily energy expenditure. If the body starts dropping muscle, it starts dropping Metabolism Advantage power.

As a result, Mark's metabolism has slowed down considerably. Because he's been eating less, his TEF and RMR have gone down. Then with his muscle loss came further metabolism loss. Finally, because he's been feeling a bit sluggish (due to the low calorie intake), he's been less active.

Mark, however, doesn't realize all this. All he knows is that he has lost 20 pounds and needs to celebrate. He "goes off" his diet and starts eating normally again. Because he's so hungry, however, he overeats on a daily basis, consuming more calories than he did before he went on the diet. This isn't gross overeating; it's just a few calories here and there that add up. Beyond that, occasionally he really over-does it and eats an entire pizza along with a plate of wings (and, of course, some beer). The weight starts coming back—and fast.

Now, you may be thinking, "So Mark's weak. I would have the discipline to control my eating. I'd go right back to my prediet food intake." Even if Mark had managed to do that, he would still have gained back the weight. Remember, since his diet has ended, he has a slower metabolism and less muscle mass, so his new calorie require-ments are even lower than they were before the diet started. His slug-gish metabolism now thinks that even his normal intake is overeating.

In the end, Mark has starved his brain and muscle, and, after stopping the diet, fed his fat. Poor Mark. He'll end up back where he started, but this time he'll have less muscle and more fat.

So what are his choices? Well, he can start the vicious cycle over again, eating progressively less until he has to "diet" for the rest of his life to keep off the weight. He can give up hope altogether, get used to being overweight, and await the inevitable consequences (including diabetes, cardiovascular disease, and increased risk of sev-eral other diseases).

Or he can do neither and, once and for all, learn how to lose weight the right way—the Metabolism Advantage way.

If you were Mark, what would you do? Well, you'd look for the Metabolism Advantage, of course. After all, you are reading this book.

Before you find out how to do just that, let's take a look at one more strategy that *won't* help you: calorie counting.

Why Calorie Counting Doesn't Work

I'm about to tell you something that's going to seem completely ludi-crous at first. To lose weight, you don't need to pay attention to how much you eat. Yes, I know, you probably think I'm off my rocker, but bear with me here.

Over the years, nutritionists have taught us to count calories. These dietitians recommend that you balance your daily energy intake with your daily energy expenditure. In other words, you eat as many calories as (or fewer than) you burn through exercise and daily life. So if you burn 3,000 calories a day, and you eat 3,000 calories that day, you'll maintain your weight and remain healthy. Of course, if you eat less, you'll lose weight. If you eat more, you'll gain weight.

It sounds great in theory, but it doesn't work so great in practice. There are four reasons for that.

1. For starters, this approach doesn't differentiate between cottage cheese and Cheez Whiz, fat-free milk and Milk Duds, apples and apple pie. Presumably, according to this approach, if you're burning 3,000 calories a day and eating 2,500 calories a day, you'd end up with the same lean body regardless of whether those calories are in the form of a balanced diet or beer and Buffalo wings. If that sounds absurd to you, it's because it *is* absurd.

2. This approach ignores the fact that different foods act differently in your body, digesting at different rates, causing the release of different hormones, affecting your ability to lose fat, and altering your ability to gain muscle.

3. Also ignored is the fact that changes in intake can impact expenditure. As I mentioned earlier, when you eat less, your metabolism slows, and then you have to eat even less. Keep restricting calories, and you end up chasing your tail all the way to a super-slow metabolic rate that's even harder to rev back up.

4. Who the heck wants to count calories all the time? And even if you did want to, you'd never truly know precisely how many calories you were burning at any given point in time. Yes, nutritionists can gauge roughly how many calories you burn a

day based on your current daily exercise and lifestyle habits, but it's only a guess. It can easily be off by 250 daily calories or more. Over a year, that discrepancy can add up to 26 pounds! If you don't know how many calories you're burning, how can you know how many to eat? You can't.

Thus, calorie counting seems like a losing proposition. This weight-loss method just doesn't add up to a faster metabolism and a lean body.

That said, don't make the mistake of thinking that how much you eat is irrelevant. It is completely relevant. If you eat too much, you'll gain weight. If you eat too little, you'll lose weight. That's how it works. For all intents and purposes, however, even if you try, you can't possibly count calories effectively enough to really know whether you're in energy balance, overeating, or undereating. In a research laboratory, calorie counting works. In real life, it doesn't.

Now, finally, let's take a look at what does work. It's time to learn how eating *more* can result in *less* body fat.

Metabolism Advantage Eating

At its core, the Metabolism Advantage nutrition plan is about dietary displacement. Dietary displacement happens when one food or combination of foods displaces other foods from your nutritional repertoire. You can eat only so much in a day, so if, for example, you eat a Big Mac and a large order of fries for lunch, you won't also eat a chicken breast and a salad. This is an example of the bad kind of dietary displacement, where unhealthful foods displace good foods.

Since much of the population of North America is using this type of bad dietary displacement, I'd like to teach you how to use good dietary displacement to your advantage. In the Metabolism Advantage plan, you'll add new and better foods to your dietary repertoire. These foods—such as lean red meat, chicken, avocado, berries, and quinoa—will displace other not-so-metabolism-friendly foods. Instead of eating a big pasta dinner, you'll have a Greek burger. Instead of eating cereal for breakfast, you'll have a Denver omelet. In the end, you'll eat more, and you'll eat better! Most important, you'll do this without even really thinking about it. By following the Metabolism Advantage rules of eating, good dietary displacement happens somewhat effortlessly.

In addition to starving fat and feeding muscle, the Metabolism Advantage approach is one that you can follow for the rest of your life. No more deprivation, no more cravings, no more binges, no more muscle loss, no more spare tire.

Now, you may be thinking, "Yeah, right. I've heard this before." You don't have to take my word for it. I challenge you to test out my bold promise by following the seven Metabolism Advantage Rules in the pages that follow. Couple them with the Metabolism Advantage supplement and exercise programs, and you'll be a believer in just 8 short weeks.

Rule #1: Eat Every 2 to 3 Hours

Each time you eat, you stimulate your metabolism for a short period of time. The TEF represents the amount of energy your body burns to digest, absorb, and either store or break down the food you eat, so the more frequently you eat, the more of a metabolic boost you'll get. If you eat only three meals a day, you get only three TEF-induced increases in metabolism. If you eat six meals a day, you boost your metabolism six times. Now that's what I call taking advantage of your metabolism.

In addition to increasing metabolism, eating every 2 to 3 hours feeds muscle and starves fat. By eating frequently, you reassure your fearful body that food is always going to be available. Your body has been encoded to fear famine and starvation. In our not-so-distant past, food wasn't as abundant as it is in North America today. The human body adapted to those scarce conditions, storing fat whenever the slightest signal of hunger or starvation became evident. It's your body's natural inclination to starve muscle and feed fat when food intake is low, infrequent, or sporadic.

If you skip breakfast, eat a small lunch, and pig out at dinner (as most North Americans do), your body starts to think that you're starving. As a result, it starts breaking down all that pesky, metabolically costly muscle and begins storing lots of fat just in case your next dinner never comes.

If you send your body the right signals, however, by eating every 2 to 3 hours, you'll get the Metabolism Advantage faster than you ever thought possible. Your body will grow progressively more comfortable feeding the muscle and starving the fat, even if another Ice Age is just around the corner.

The ramifications of this simple Metabolism Advantage rule really add up. According to research from Georgia State University, people who eat every 2 to 3 hours (versus eating only two or three meals each day) have better blood sugar levels, fewer stress and muscle-breakdown hormones, more muscle-building hormones, less blood cholesterol, and most important for you, less body fat and higher metabolic rates.

At this point, the one thought on your mind should be: "Isn't it about time for a meal?"

Rule #2: Build with Protein

Now that you know *how often* to eat, let's talk about *what* to eat. Most people automatically assume that when I say eat every 2 to 3 hours, I must be talking about "little feedings"—snacks and so forth. This isn't what I mean at all. I want every feeding to be complete. You don't have to eat huge meals, but you shouldn't feel as if you're eating bird feed, either. Every 2 to 3 hours, you want to focus on building a complete meal according to the rules you'll learn in this book. To build a complete meal, you'll start with protein. In fact, every one of your daily meals and snacks should include protein, for the following reasons.

- **Increased TEF.** Your body burns calories to digest, absorb, and store all macronutrients (proteins, carbohydrates, and fats). That said, the thermic effect of protein is roughly double that of carbohydrates and fat. Therefore, including protein in your meals and snacks will boost your metabolism during digestion all day long.

- **Increased fat-loss hormones.** Eating protein leads to the release of glucagon, a hormone that helps coax fat out of your fat cells so it can be burned up by your muscles. It also makes your fat cells less receptive to storing fat.

- **Increased muscle building.** Your muscles are made up of protein. When you work out hard—as you will on the Metabolism Advantage exercise plan—you need a little extra dietary protein to help make them bigger and stronger. In fact, studies completed by William Evans, PhD, at the University of Arkansas for Medical Sciences, have demonstrated that "the RDA for protein (the typically recommended amount) may not be adequate to completely meet the metabolic and physiological needs of virtually all older people."

- **Reduced cardiovascular risk.** Several studies conducted at the University of Western Ontario in Canada have shown that increasing the percentage of protein in the diet (from 11 percent to 23 percent) while decreasing the percentage of carbohydrate (from 63 percent to 48 percent) lowers bad (LDL) cholesterol and triglycerides while increasing good (HDL) cholesterol concentrations.

- **Improved weight loss.** According to research at the University of Illinois, elevating daily protein intake increases body fat loss, spares muscle mass, reduces triglycerides, decreases feelings of hunger, and improves blood sugar. These studies have also demonstrated that eating high-quality protein at breakfast may even further supercharge the fat-loss process.

- **Improved overall nutrition.** We don't eat just protein; we eat food. Therefore, higher-protein foods often contain other nutrients that enhance health, body composition, and performance. These nutrients include iron, B vitamins, creatine, branched-chain amino acids, and conjugated linoleic acids.

With all of those benefits, it should come as no surprise that on the Metabolism Advantage plan, you're going to eat protein every 2 to 3 hours.

Rule #3: Balance with Veggies

If protein is your super builder, veggies are its sidekick. Simply put, don't eat one without the other. Since you'll eat protein every 2 to 3 hours, you'll also eat veggies every 2 to 3 hours. Aw, come on. No whining. In the Metabolism Advantage recipes in Chapter 8, you'll find many interesting and tasty ways to get more veggies into your diet. First, however, let's talk about why you're going to eat veggies with each meal.

Veggies balance your body's pH. You probably think of test tubes and beakers when you think of pH, but your blood, bones, and organs all function optimally at a certain pH. Without getting too scientific, pH stands for "potential of hydrogen." Your body's pH represents the balance of positively charged (acid-forming) ions to

COVERING YOUR DIETARY BASES

Use this chart to determine which foods are acid producing, which foods are base producing, and which are neutral. If you can't find a certain food on the list, it probably has the same status as the other foods in its category. For example, mangos aren't on the list, but since they're fruits, they're probably base producing. Likewise, cashews aren't on the list, but since they're nuts, they're probably acid producing.

ACID PRODUCERS

MEATS	GRAINS	DAIRY
Beef, lean	Brown rice	Buttermilk
Chicken	Cornflakes	Cheddar cheese, low-fat
Corned beef, canned	Egg noodles	Cottage cheese
Frankfurters	Mixed grain rye bread	Fruit yogurt, low-fat, lactose-free
Liver sausage	Mixed grain wheat bread	Gouda cheese
Lunchmeat	Oats	Hard cheese
Pork, lean	Rye bread	Ice cream
Rump steak	Rye crackers	Parmesan cheese
Salami	Rye flour	Plain yogurt, low-fat, lactose-free
Turkey	Wheat bread	Processed cheese
Veal fillet	Wheat flour	Sour cream
EGGS	White bread	Whole milk
FISH	White rice	**NUTS**
Cod fillet	White spaghetti	Peanuts
Haddock	Whole grain spaghetti	Walnuts
Herring		**LEGUMES**
Trout		Lentils
		Peas
		DRINKS
		Beer, pale
		Coca-Cola

negatively charged (alkalinizing) ions. When you eat more acidic foods without balancing them out with more alkaline foods, you suffer a host of ill consequences, including a sluggish metabolism.

Each component of every food you eat will, after digestion and absorption, present itself to the kidneys as either an acid-forming compound or a base-forming one. One common problem with our

BASE PRODUCERS

VEGETABLES	FRUITS	SWEETS
Asparagus	Apple juice	Honey
Broccoli	Apples	Marmalade
Carrots	Apricots	Sugar
Cauliflower	Bananas	**DRINKS**
Celery	Black currants	Beer, draft
Chicory	Cherries	Beer, stout
Cucumber	Grape juice	Cocoa
Eggplant	Kiwifruit	Coffee
Green beans	Lemon juice	Mineral water
Leeks	Orange juice	Tea
Lettuce	Oranges	Wine, red
Mushrooms	Peaches	Wine, white
Onions	Pears	
Peppers	Pineapple	
Potatoes	Raisins	
Radishes	Strawberries	
Spinach	Watermelon	
Tomato juice		
Tomatoes		
Zucchini		

NEUTRAL

FATS AND OILS

Butter
Margarine
Olive oil
Sunflower oil

SOURCE: Adapted from T. Remer and F. Manz, "Potential Renal Acid Load of Foods and Its Influence on pH." *Journal of the American Dietetic Association*, 95, no. 7 (1995): 791–97. For more foods and their relative values, visit www.MetabolismAdvantage.com.

North American diet is that it produces mostly acids and few bases. Like any type of excess, this throws off the delicate balance inside the body.

Your body does everything it can to maintain a blood pH of about 7.4. To do so, it deposits and withdraws alkalinizing minerals and other substances from other body tissues as needed. When you eat a

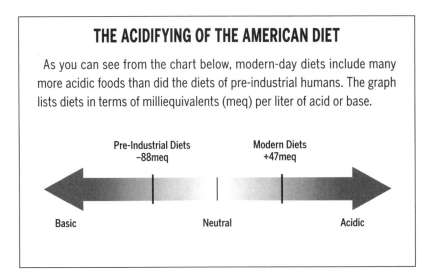

THE ACIDIFYING OF THE AMERICAN DIET

As you can see from the chart below, modern-day diets include many more acidic foods than did the diets of pre-industrial humans. The graph lists diets in terms of milliequivalents (meq) per liter of acid or base.

Pre-Industrial Diets
−88meq

Modern Diets
+47meq

Basic   Neutral   Acidic

highly acidic diet with few bases and force your body to repeatedly steal alkalinizing substances from various tissues, you set off a cascade of consequences that include:

- An increase in muscle-breakdown hormones (cortisol)
- A decrease in muscle-building hormones (growth hormone and IGF-1)
- A decrease in metabolic boost (thyroid hormone)
- A loss of bone mass (osteoporosis) as the minerals from your bones are used to lower the pH of your blood
- A loss of muscle mass

And the situation only worsens as you age. Once you get older, your kidneys don't work as well and, as a result, you can't handle acids as well. In fact, some scientists think that the muscle and bone loss associated with aging may be caused by a chronically high-acid diet.

Veggies are the great acid neutralizers, among the best alkalinizing foods around. This is why protein and veggies are necessary bedmates. Proteins have a lot to offer, but even the leanest types are quite acidic. Partner your high-protein foods with veggies, however, and you've got the ultimate combo that boosts your metabolism, neutralizes acid, strengthens bones, and encourages muscle growth. So every meal you eat—even if it's just a snack—must contain some lean protein and a heaping serving of veggies.

For more information about dietary acids and bases, visit www.MetabolismAdvantage.com.

Veggies contain fiber. Fiber is a critical nutrient for optimal health and body composition. It literally gums up the digestive process, slowing the passage of carbohydrates into the bloodstream. This helps stabilize blood sugar levels, which in turn helps stabilize your energy levels and appetite. Fiber passes through your intestine largely undigested, sucking some other foods—and their calories—along with it. Fiber also lowers your risk of certain cancers and heart disease. Although the government recommends we consume 25 to 35 grams per day, most of us eat less than half that amount.

Veggies have antioxidants. Antioxidants soak up those nasty free radicals that accumulate in your body as a result of exposure to unavoidable environmental chemicals, food preservatives, and cigarette smoke and as a side effect of normal aerobic metabolism. Free radicals wreak havoc on all the cells of your body, including the all-important mitochondria that run your metabolism.

Although your body makes its own antioxidants, certain foods, including vegetables, offer additional antioxidant protection. Eat a diet rich in these foods, and you can expect a plentiful supply of vitamins and minerals as well as an increase in your body's total antioxidant power. By powering up your antioxidant status, you can reduce some of the effects of aging, including memory loss, blood vessel damage, and plaque buildup in your arteries. You'll also experience less damage to your genetic material, DNA.

Veggies have phytochemicals. *Phytochemicals* (or sometimes *phytonutrients*) is a fancy word for the nutritional content of fruits and veggies (and some other foods, such as whole grains) that isn't easily categorized. Phytochemicals are not vitamins, and they're not minerals. They are not fiber or fat or protein or carbohydrate. They are

THE BEST ANTIOXIDANT FOODS

Although the nutritional supplement industry has gone crazy promoting antioxidant formulas, the best (and cheapest, I might add) antioxidants come from plain old fruits and veggies. The following chart presents vegetables and fruits rich in antioxidant power. The higher the number, the greater the ability to soak up free radicals. If you want to rev up your metabolism, you should eat a few foods from each list every day. The foods listed in bold type are included regularly in the Metabolism Advantage menus.

VEGETABLE	ANTIOXIDANT POWER	FRUIT	ANTIOXIDANT POWER
Kale	1,770	Prunes	5,770
Spinach, raw	1,260	Raisins	2,830
Brussels sprouts	980	**Blueberries**	2,400
Alfalfa sprouts	930	**Blackberries**	2,036
Spinach, steamed	909	**Cranberries**	1,750
Broccoli florets	890	**Strawberries**	1,540
Beets	841	**Raspberries**	1,220
Red bell pepper	713	Plums	949
		Oranges	750
		Red grapes	739

SOURCE: Adapted from J. McBride, "High ORAC Foods May Slow Aging." *Agriculture Research*, February 8, 1999. (1 serving = 100 g or 3.5 oz)

simply chemicals that plants make, usually in the form of pigments, to enhance their survival. These chemicals fend off attacks from bugs and other pests and help plants survive drought and other extreme weather conditions. Many of these chemicals have been shown to improve human health as well. For example, a phytochemical called lycopene, found in tomatoes, has been shown to reduce the growth of cancer cells. Red wine (and red grapes) contain other phytochemicals called polyphenols that may reduce the risk of heart disease and cancer.

Although the nutritional supplement industry has done a fantastic job of isolating, extracting, and packaging many of these phytochemicals in pill form, the best (and cheapest) phytochemicals come from fruits and vegetables.

Rule #4: Eat Most Types of Carbs after Exercise

Although low-carb and high-carb diets are constantly duking it out for nutritional supremacy, both types work—some of the time. You see, your body handles carbohydrates differently at different times of the day. That's why people seem to get some results with each type of program. You don't have to avoid carbs or, alternatively, load up on them to get results, though. You just have to know when your body best tolerates certain types of carbs. Then you can eat them when your body wants them and avoid them when it doesn't. This concept is called nutrient timing, and with it, you can literally have your cake and eat it, too.

You may know that there are different types of proteins and different types of fats. There are also different types of carbs, which have different properties in your body.

Now, some people in the nutrition community would have you believe that some of these types of carbs—quickly digested, refined foods—are bad for you *all the time*, whereas other types—fiber-rich, whole grain foods—are good for you *all the time*. This just isn't the case. In fact, some refined, quickly digested carbs are good for your metabolism at some times and not at others. The same holds true for high-fiber whole grains.

Really, the answer to this confusing debate is this: Some carbs are really good for you some of the time, and others are really bad for you some of the time. As an old nutrition professor once said to me, "There's no such thing as a good or bad food. Rather, there are only good and bad times to eat certain foods."

Therefore, you just have to know when your body best tolerates certain carbs and eat the right ones at the right times.

There are three main types of carbohydrates.

1. **Fiber-rich carbs.** These vegetables and fruits house plenty of fiber to slow the absorption of carbohydrates into your system. They provide slow, even rises in blood sugar, which controls

THE BEST TIMES TO EAT CARBS

Consult the chart below to find out when to eat each of the three main types of carbohydrates.

CARBOHYDRATE TYPE	EXAMPLE FOODS	MOST APPROPRIATE TIME TO EAT
Fibrous	Beans Legumes Some fruits Vegetables	Any time of day (especially for vegetables)
Starchy	Breads Cereal grains Pasta Potatoes Whole grains	During the 3 hours after exercise
Sugars	Desserts Fruit juices Many processed food additives Sodas Sports drinks Table sugar	Only during and/or immediately after exercise

hunger and blood sugar levels. These foods are also micronutrient dense. You can eat many of these wholesome carbs—specifically vegetables and fruits low in sugar—at any time of day.

2. **Starchy carbohydrates.** Cereal, rice, bread, and potatoes are carbohydrate dense and offer less micronutrition for every calorie you consume than do fiber-rich carbs. This doesn't make these foods inherently bad for you, but it does mean you need to watch your intake. The best time to eat these carbs is during the few hours after exercise. It's during this time period that your muscle cells open their doors to starchy carbohydrates. After exercise, your body stores carbs as muscle glycogen, burning fat as its primary fuel source. During other times of the day, your muscles are not as receptive, and as a result, these types of carbs can eventually wind up in places you don't want them, such as your fat cells.

3. **Refined sugars.** These foods are typically considered empty

calories. They have lots in the way of carbs but little in the way of vitamins, minerals, and phytochemicals. That said, they aren't bad for you *all the time*, as some people would lead you to believe. You can eat these foods during and immediately after exercise. During this critical time period, these carbs give your body quick energy for recovery. If you haven't just finished exercising, though, put down the Twinkies!

Rule #5: Balance Your Fats

Fat is really bad for you, right? Or is it good for you? Hmm, this is starting to sound like the same dilemma you had with carbohydrates.

Well, having learned what you have so far, you can probably guess what I'm going to say next. That's right, there are different types of fats, all with different properties in your body.

The appropriate use of dietary fat, contrary to most people's beliefs, can actually help you lose body fat. You see, in your body, dietary fat is responsible for the control of inflammation as well as cell composition, blood fat profile, the ability to handle carbohydrates, heart disease risk, and body composition. To improve your body and your health, it's important to get a good balance of the three different types of dietary fats—saturated, monounsaturated, and polyunsaturated.

That said, most people are out of balance. Just as most of us eat too many acidic foods—putting our pH off-balance—we also tend to eat too many of the wrong types of fats, which creates its own form of imbalance in the body. Certain types of fat—such as the omega-3 fatty acids found in salmon and flaxseed—help to reduce levels of pro-inflammatory hormones called cytokines. Omega-6 fatty acids—found in many cooking oils—tend to raise levels of these very hormones. Now, when you eat omega-3 fats and omega-6 fats in balance, you end up with balanced levels of inflammatory hormones. Most people, however, eat far too many omega-6s and far too few omega-

HOW MUCH FAT?

Use this chart to help you get the right balance of fats every day.

FAT TYPE	EXAMPLE FOODS	HOW MUCH SHOULD BE IN YOUR DIET
Saturated	Any animal food, such as beef, pork, eggs, butter, and milk (coconut oil is one of the vegetable exceptions)	About $\frac{1}{3}$ of total fat intake
Monounsaturated	Avocados Nuts and nut butters Olive oil	About $\frac{1}{3}$ of total fat intake
Polyunsaturated	Fish oils Flaxseed Nuts and nut butters Vegetable oils	About $\frac{1}{3}$ of total fat intake (with about 50 percent from omega-3 fats and 50 percent from omega-6 fats)

3s. This sets the stage for inflammation throughout the body, causing joint pain, heart disease, and muscle loss.

That's right. Researchers have linked high levels of inflammation to high levels of catabolic hormones in muscles. These hormones *break down* muscle protein.

According to research, optimal body function (including fat loss) requires a good amount of total fats as well as a healthy balance of the three types of fat: one-third saturated, one-third monounsaturated, and one-third polyunsaturated. The Metabolism Advantage plan includes precisely this balance. Consuming the right types of fats in the right amounts doesn't have to be complicated. Simply be sure that each day, you eat some saturated fat, some monounsaturated fat, and some polyunsaturated fat. Use the chart above to guide your eating.

Rule #6: Eat These Foods Every Week

As I've mentioned, if you eat protein with each meal, your metabolism will rev right up. Save carbs for after exercise, and you'll feed your muscle and not your fat. Eat the right fats, and you'll prevent disease while dropping body fat.

But, as my old nutrition professor used to say, we don't eat proteins, carbohydrates, and fats. We eat food! We eat apples and chicken and fish and oatmeal. So rather than leave you with just a few general macronutrient rules, let's take a look at which foods should be on your plan—the Metabolism Advantage Metafoods.

The Metabolism Advantage Metafoods are the best metabolism-boosting, fat-stripping, muscle-building, age-defying foods available. Once you've incorporated these foods into your diet, you'll automatically stop eating the "other" foods. Think about it: If most of your meals are filled with these good foods, you won't have much time or appetite for others.

I've carefully selected the Metabolism Advantage Metafoods for the following reasons.

1. They are nutrient dense, containing the most micronutrient, fiber, and phytochemical bang for your buck. These Metafoods provide more metabolism-boosting, muscle-building, fat-burning, and anti-aging benefits than another food containing the same number of calories.
2. These foods easily fit into the delicious meal plan outlined in Chapter 8. Whoever said eating well had to be bland, boring, or depressing? I certainly didn't!
3. You can find these foods at most supermarkets or health food stores.

So without further ado, here are the Metabolism Advantage Metafoods.

Lean red meat (top round, sirloin, or 96% lean ground beef). Red meat is full of B vitamins, heme iron (the most absorbable form of iron), conjugated linoleic acid (CLA, a fat-burning fatty acid), and creatine (for muscle building).

Salmon. Salmon has both protein and omega-3 fatty acids, a dynamic duo that leads to increased fat burning. At this point, you should know all too well that protein does a great job of revving your metabolism. According to a recent study, the right amount of the kind of omega-3 fats found in fish oil can boost your metabolism by a whopping 400 calories each day. It does this while fighting diabetes, heart disease, and cancer.

Omega-3 eggs. Produced by hens that eat a diet rich in flaxseed, these eggs offer benefits similar to those of salmon. They pack a one-two protein and omega-3 punch. Don't fear the yolks—that's where you'll find the omega-3s. Available brands include Pilgrim's Pride Eggs Plus and Eggland's Best.

Low-fat, lactose-free plain yogurt. Yogurt is a smooth and creamy way to boost the protein content of your diet. Eat yogurt, and you also get some great calcium. Research from the University of Tennessee shows that increased calcium consumption speeds metabolism and promotes fat loss. That's right, this mineral isn't just for bones and teeth.

Spinach. Spinach is a great base-producing food. A spinach salad or some cooked spinach can neutralize nearly any acid-forming food, and that's good for your bones and muscles. Spinach also contains fiber to improve gastrointestinal health and promote fat loss. And it has folate, which reduces the risk of heart disease, cancer, and age-related memory loss. Popeye was right—you'd better eats your spinach!

Tomatoes. In addition to tasting delicious, tomatoes are full of fiber and vitamin C. Cooked tomatoes (even those in tomato sauce) are also rich in lycopene. Increasing your lycopene intake will let you enjoy a 50 percent reduction in heart disease and prostate cancer risk.

Cruciferous vegetables (broccoli, cabbage, cauliflower). These veggies contain a special class of nutrients called indoles that have been found to reduce the risk of a variety of cancers, balance hormone status, and offer antioxidant benefits. When Mother Nature made these veggies, she added some fiber for good measure.

Avocados. Avocados are actually fruits, not vegetables. Surprised? Well, how about this: Avocados are probably the healthiest fruits on the block. They contain a heaping portion of B vitamins, fiber, folate, and zinc (among other nutrients). Zinc is particularly important for men since it's involved in testosterone production. Eat your avocados, and your sex life might get a boost! Finally, these fruits are also rich in monounsaturated fats.

Mixed berries. Strawberries, blueberries, raspberries, and other types of berries have huge amounts of antioxidant power. In fact, berries rank high in their ability to soak up those nasty, cell-damaging free radicals.

Oranges. Oranges are best known for what? Their vitamin C content, of course. But they also happen to be great sources of fiber and folate.

Mixed beans (kidney beans, black beans, and chickpeas). One cup of beans provides a whopping 11 grams of fiber. In addition, beans keep your blood sugar low, controlling diabetes. Finally, and interestingly, several studies now show that eating beans can add years to your life. If you soak dried beans overnight with a small amount of baking soda, they won't make you so gassy.

Quinoa. This is truly a supergrain. The Incas looked to this grain to make them strong for work and battle, and they had good reason. Quinoa is rich in a variety of vitamins and minerals, such as calcium, magnesium, iron, phosphorus, and B vitamins. In addition, it is one of the only grains that provide complete protein—all of the amino acids your muscles need for growth. Finally, since quinoa contains no gluten, it's the best grain for people who have gastrointestinal problems related to wheat allergies.

Whole oats (large flake). Oats and quinoa run neck and neck for the title of healthiest grain, so make sure you include both in your diet. Like quinoa, oats also control blood sugar. They are also rich in the B vitamins and vitamin E, are a hypoallergenic relative of wheat and other grains, and contain more soluble fiber than any other grain.

Mixed nuts. Although nuts used to be considered bad news because of their fat content, we now know that they're among the healthiest foods around. Eating nuts regularly has been shown to decrease the risk of several diseases (including heart disease) and to promote weight loss. This is due to the fact that nuts are rich in dietary fiber, magnesium, copper, folate, potassium, and vitamin E. They're also loaded with healthy polyunsaturated and monounsaturated fats that speed up metabolism. Since different nuts have different ratios of fatty acids, your best bet is to eat a mixture.

Olive oil. In addition to revving up your metabolism, the monounsaturated fats found in olive oil help reduce the risk of all sorts of diseases. Prepare your meals with olive oil and pretend you're dining on the coast of the Mediterranean.

Flaxseed and flaxseed oil. These products contain the heart-healthy omega-3 fatty acids. As I've mentioned, these oils have been shown to boost metabolism, increase muscle building, decrease disease risk, improve intelligence, and reduce depression. In women, they've even been shown to reduce the symptoms of menopause.

Green tea. There's an old Chinese saying that goes, "Better to go without food for a week than without green tea for a day." The Chinese were on to something. Green tea offers a host of benefits, including cancer prevention, fat loss, improved blood sugar, and better blood circulation. Live longer and better by drinking your green tea! (You'll learn more about the benefits of green tea in Chapter 4.)

Make it your goal to eat most of these Metafoods three to five times each week. The meal plan in Chapter 8 will offer these foods every week for 8 weeks, making them a regular habit.

Rule #7: Eat the Right Foods at the Right Times

You've already learned a little about nutrient timing in our discussion of carbohydrates, but I have even more for you to digest on this topic. Now remember, the most critical nutrient-timing concept is this: What you eat is determined by when you work out. During and after workouts, you want protein and carbs but little fat. During the rest of the day, you want proteins, good fats, and veggies. Here's a closer look at how it works, based on the main categories of foods and supplements you'll be taking in on the Metabolism Advantage plan.

Whole food protein. In every meal, you should eat a lean source of protein, such as lean meat, fish, yogurt, or omega-3 eggs.

Supplemental protein. You'll use a protein powder when you make the various types of Super Shakes on the Metabolism Advantage plan. These powders provide a nice metabolism boost when you can't have a whole food source.

Not all supplemental proteins are created equal. Whey protein isolate is quickly digested and best consumed during and immediately after exercise (as part of your liquid recovery supplement). Casein protein isolate and milk protein isolates (whey and casein) are slower to digest and are best consumed outside of the workout and post-workout periods. You'll learn more about protein supplements in Chapter 4.

Vegetables and fruits. You should eat spinach, tomatoes, avocados, berries, oranges, and other low-sugar fruits and vegetables with every meal to balance your protein consumption. Although you can

EATING BY THE 90 PERCENT RULE

You need not follow the Metabolism Advantage nutrition plan 100 percent of the time. As long as you follow it 90 percent of the time, you'll still get great results.

What does 90 percent translate into in terms of real food? Let's do the math. Since you're going to eat about six meals a day, 7 days a week, you'll have 42 feeding opportunities each week. Ten percent of that is 4.2 meals. Therefore, you're allowed to deviate from the Metabolism Advantage nutrition plan four times each week (although most people are so satisfied by the plan that they deviate even less).

Now, these approved deviations do not include downing an entire pizza followed by a full box of Krispy Kremes. Rather, they include some foods, in reasonable quantities, that might not normally fit into the Metabolism Advantage plan.

For example, you might eat a couple slices of pizza on a Saturday evening, enjoy a piece of cheesecake after dinner on Sunday, drink a beer or glass of wine after work on Wednesday, or have some chocolate on Monday morning.

Just be careful here. Make sure your 10 percent doesn't become 20 percent or 30 percent. If you're eating 42 meals a week, you're allowed to eat 4 meals or snacks per week that aren't part of the Metabolism Advantage program—and that's all. The best way to make sure you don't go overboard is to schedule your 10 percent meals. Pick a day and a meal and schedule it just as you schedule your exercise days. This will keep you committed to your eating plan as well as let you look forward to something different. Of course, if you simply must have one of your 10 percent meals outside of its regularly scheduled time, go for it. Just make sure you don't double up. Cross the planned 10 percent meal off your schedule.

eat all the vegetables you want at any time of day, be careful about how much fruit you load onto your plate outside the workout window. One piece of fruit, such as an orange or apple, is fine with breakfast even if you're working out in the afternoon. On the other hand, eating an entire bunch of grapes—which are high in fruit sugar—will probably flood your body with too much carbohydrate outside the workout window. So if you're going to eat a lot of fruit, save much of it for the postworkout period. It's during this time that your body best tolerates higher-carbohydrate foods.

Starches, grains, and sugars. Save foods such as quinoa, whole oats, pasta, whole grains, rice, and sugar for during and after exercise, when your muscles are most receptive to burning these carbs for fuel or storing them for later use. Here's a simple rule: If you have not exercised within the past hours, put away the bread, pasta, oats, cereals, and so on. Even postworkout, most of your carbs should come from the super sources quinoa and whole oats.

Fats. The best time to eat fats is the opposite of the best time to eat starchy and grainy carbohydrates. Have nuts, olive oil, fish oil, flaxseed, flaxseed oil, egg yolks, and fat from meats and dairy outside the postexercise period. Make sure you sample evenly from the three main fat sources—and especially from the foods listed among the Metabolism Advantage Metafoods discussed in Rule #6.

Recovery drinks. Recovery drinks contain fast-digesting protein and sugar. Although sugar isn't the best selection during most of the day, a recovery drink is just what the exercise doctor ordered during and immediately after workouts. During these times, your body repairs itself best with this type of drink. As with protein supplements, you'll learn more about these drinks in Chapter 4.

To make things even simpler for you, starting on page 70, I've assembled a sample day's worth of meals for various workout situations. This will give you an at-a-glance peek at exactly how to time your nutrient intake based on the time of day you work out. Let's start with the morning folks.

The Morning Workout

■ **6:00 TO 7:00 AM: WORKOUT** ▪ Meal of fast-digesting protein and carbs

Sip ½ recovery drink

■ **7:00 AM: POSTWORKOUT SNACK** ▪ Meal of fast-digesting protein and carbs

Sip other ½ recovery drink

■ **8:30 AM: BREAKFAST** ▪ Since it's postexercise, you can build your meal around protein, veggies, and carbohydrates like oatmeal and berries

4 egg whites with 1 omega-3 egg, spinach, and tomato
1 serving oatmeal and frozen mixed berries
1 cup green tea

■ **NOON: LUNCH** ▪ Since your workout was 5 hours ago, this meal should be higher in protein, fat, and veggies and lower in carbs

1 piece salmon
Spinach salad made with broccoli, avocado, tomatoes, carrots, and mixed nuts, with flaxseed oil and olive oil dressing
2 fish-oil capsules (more on these in Chapter 4)

■ **3:00 PM: MIDAFTERNOON SNACK** ▪ Since your workout was hours ago, have a snack low in carbs and built around protein and fruits/veggies

Super Shake
    1 cup iced green tea
    1 scoop milk protein blend
    3 tablespoons low-fat, lactose-free plain yogurt
    ½ cup frozen mixed berries
    1 serving Greens+ (more on this supplement in Chapter 4)
2 fish-oil capsules

■ **6:00 PM: DINNER** ▪ Since it's been many hours since your workout, have a dinner low in carbs and built around protein and fruits/veggies

Extra-lean (96%) ground beef burger
Spinach salad made with broccoli, avocado, tomatoes, carrots, and mixed beans, with flaxseed oil and olive oil dressing

■ **9:30 PM: EVENING SNACK** ▪ Since your workout was hours ago, have a snack low in carbs and built around protein and fruits/veggies

Super Shake
    1 cup iced green tea
    1 scoop milk protein blend

3 tablespoons low-fat, lactose-free plain yogurt
½ cup frozen mixed berries
1 serving Greens+
2 fish-oil capsules

The Afternoon Workout

■ **7:00 AM: BREAKFAST** ▪ **You haven't worked out yet, so this meal should be higher in protein, fat, and veggies and lower in carbs**

4 egg whites with 2 omega-3 eggs, spinach, feta cheese, and tomato
1 orange
2 fish-oil capsules
1 cup green tea

■ **10:00 AM: MIDMORNING SNACK** ▪ **You still haven't worked out, so have a snack low in carbs and built around protein and fruits/veggies**

Super Shake
1 cup iced green tea
1 scoop milk protein blend
3 tablespoons low-fat, lactose-free plain yogurt
½ cup frozen mixed berries
1 serving Greens+
2 fish-oil capsules

■ **NOON TO 1:00 PM: WORKOUT** ▪ **Meal of fast-digesting protein and carbs**

Sip ½ recovery drink

■ **1:00 PM: POSTWORKOUT SNACK** ▪ **Meal of fast-digesting protein and carbs**

Sip other ½ recovery drink

■ **3:00 PM: MIDAFTERNOON SNACK** ▪ **Since it's postexercise, you can build your meal around protein, veggies, and carbohydrates like quinoa and fruits**

Meat loaf made with extra-lean (96%) ground beef, quinoa,
    and omega-3 egg whites
Sautéed spinach, onions, olive oil, and tomatoes
1 orange
1 cup green tea

■ **6:00 PM: DINNER** ▪ Since your workout was 5 hours ago, this meal should be higher in protein, fat, and veggies and lower in carbs

> *1 piece salmon*
> *Spinach salad made with broccoli, avocado, tomatoes, carrots, mixed*
> *beans, flaxseed oil and olive oil dressing*

■ **9:30 PM: EVENING SNACK** ▪ Since your workout was hours ago, have a snack low in carbs and built around protein and fruits/veggies

> *Super Shake*
> *1 cup iced green tea*
> *1 scoop milk protein blend*
> *3 tablespoons low-fat, lactose-free plain yogurt*
> *½ cup frozen mixed berries*
> *1 serving Greens+*
> *2 fish-oil capsules*

Evening Workout

■ **7:00 AM: BREAKFAST** ▪ You haven't worked out yet, so this meal should be higher in protein, fat, and veggies and lower in carbs

> *4 egg whites with 2 omega-3 eggs, spinach, feta cheese, and tomato*
> *1 orange*
> *2 fish-oil capsules*
> *1 cup green tea*

■ **10:00 AM: MIDMORNING SNACK** ▪ You still haven't worked out, so have a snack low in carbs and built around protein and fruits/veggies

> *Super Shake*
> *1 cup iced green tea*
> *1 scoop milk protein blend*
> *3 tablespoons low-fat, lactose-free plain yogurt*
> *½ cup frozen mixed berries*
> *1 serving Greens+*
> *2 fish-oil capsules*

■ **NOON: LUNCH** ▪ Since you haven't worked out yet, this meal should be higher in protein, fat, and veggies and lower in carbs

> *1 piece salmon*
> *Spinach salad made with broccoli, avocado, tomatoes, carrots, mixed*
> *nuts, flaxseed oil and olive oil dressing*
> *2 fish-oil capsules*

■ **3:00 PM: MIDAFTERNOON SNACK** ▪ Since you still haven't worked out, have a snack low in carbs and built around protein and fruits/veggies

> *Super Shake*
> *1 cup iced green tea*
> *1 scoop milk protein blend*
> *3 tablespoons low-fat, lactose-free plain yogurt*
> *½ cup frozen mixed berries*
> *1 serving Greens+*
> *2 fish-oil capsules*

■ **6:00 TO 7:00 PM: WORKOUT** ▪ Meal of fast-digesting protein and carbs

> *Sip ½ recovery drink*

■ **7:00 PM: POSTWORKOUT SNACK** ▪ Meal of fast-digesting protein and carbs

> *Sip other ½ recovery drink*

■ **9:00 PM: DINNER** ▪ Since it's postexercise, you can build your meal around protein, veggies, and carbohydrates like quinoa and fruits

> *Meat loaf made with extra lean (96%) ground beef, quinoa,*
> *and omega-3 egg whites*
> *Sautéed spinach, onions, olive oil, and tomatoes*
> *1 orange*
> *1 cup green tea*

7 Simple Rules

If you follow the seven simple nutritional rules laid out in this chapter, you'll take care of all of your nutritional needs. I don't mean to sound like a broken record, but these rules are so important they bear repeating.

1. Eat every 2 to 3 hours.
2. Eat lean protein with each meal.
3. Eat veggies with each meal.
4. Eat carbs other than fruits and veggies only during exercise and within 3 hours afterward.
5. Balance your daily fat intake among saturated, monounsaturated, and polyunsaturated fats.
6. Eat several servings of Metafoods each week.
7. Eat the right foods at the right times.

Are you:

- Eating enough food to prevent metabolic slowdown and muscle loss? Check.
- Getting enough protein? Check.
- Getting enough veggies? Check.
- Eating your carbs at the times they're best used by the body for energy and muscle restoration? Check.
- Eating enough of the right fats to reduce your risks of disease? Check.
- Eating the best foods on the planet? Check.

It's all covered here: seven simple strategies that yield great results every time. No calorie counting, no low carb, no low fat, no points, and no degree in biochemistry required.

4

The Metabolism Advantage Supplement Plan

Five essentials that will kick your metabolism
into high gear—and improve your health

The Metabolism Advantage supplement plan supports the Metabolism Advantage nutrition and exercise plans. As I've mentioned before, you can think of the supplement plan as the third leg of a three-legged stool. You need all three legs to support the stool. Take one away, and the stool collapses.

Too often, people try to get along without one or two of the three legs. They exercise without changing their diet. They take supplements without exercising. They eat less and do nothing else. Such tactics do just one thing: They take you in a frustrating circle back to where you started!

Let's say you decide to take fat-burning supplements but not to exercise or eat right. Well, many of these supplements work by coaxing your fat cells to release their cargo, so the fat leaves its usual home—the fat cell—and floats around in your blood. Since you didn't change your diet and are not exercising, that fat has nowhere else to go. Your muscles don't need it. Your organs don't need it. So you know what happens? It makes its way into another fat cell.

Let's say you change your diet, but you don't exercise. As I've mentioned before, you'll lose some weight, but you'll also lose some muscle and consequently slow your metabolism. Eventually, you'll gain back the weight.

What happens if you exercise and eat right, but you don't take the right supplements? You don't get from point A to point B as quickly. You also may miss out on some essential nutritional support. Although the media have done an effective job of convincing people that all supplements are bad news, this just isn't the case. You'll soon learn about five important supplements that everyone—men and women, thirty-somethings and baby boomers—should take to improve muscle mass, rev up metabolism, and shed fat. Yes, folks, they are that effective. Repeated studies have proven that not only are these supplements *not* bad for your health, most of them will *improve* your health. They will harmonize with your nutrition and exercise plans to produce the fastest, healthiest, and most impressive results.

The Five Essentials

In the pages that follow, you're going to learn about five nutritional supplements that are essential in your quest. These supplements will provide important muscle-building and fat-burning nutrients that are nearly impossible to consume from food alone. I take these supplements every day. So does every single one of my clients. Repeated studies done in prestigious sports nutrition labs throughout the world show that the following supplements work. They boost metabolism, stimulate fat burning, and set the stage for muscle growth. They also provide wonderful side effects, such as better blood sugar levels, reduced blood cholesterol levels, increased energy, stronger bones, and improved memory. Simply put, these nutrients have repeatedly been shown to offer benefits in terms of health, body composition, and performance outcomes.

FISH-OIL CAPSULES

Type "fish oil supplementation" into the world's largest scientific database (www.pubmed.com), and you'll find more than 1,700 scientific studies. The results of most of these studies are crystal clear: Fish-oil supplementation is a must for nearly everyone.

Fish-oil supplements have been shown to have powerful antioxidant, anti-cancer, anti-inflammatory, and anti–heart disease properties. In addition, they've been shown to improve carbohydrate tolerance and fat burning. Finally, eicosapentaenoic acid (EPA) and docosahexaenoic acid (DHA)—the omega-3 fatty acids found only in fish oil—can dramatically boost your metabolism. By dramatic, I'm talking about 400 calories a day! That's roughly the number of calories in a McDonald's double cheeseburger.

Here's how it works. The cells in your body have two main metabolic engines, the mitochondrion and the peroxisome. In Chapter 1, you learned about the importance of the mitochondrion, the main calorie-burning furnace of every cell in your body. Although not as powerful as the mitochondrion, the peroxisome burns quite a few calories, too. Fish oil increases levels of important enzymes that in turn boost the calorie-burning ability of both cell furnaces, encouraging them to waste some calories as heat. When University of Western Ontario researchers asked people to take fish-oil capsules every day for 3 weeks, the participants experienced a 400-calorie-per-day boost in metabolism.

In addition to boosting calorie burning, this supplement sets the stage for fat burning and muscle growth, both of which help boost your overall metabolic rate. Fish oil increases levels of fat-burning enzymes and decreases levels of fat-storage enzymes in your body. Also, studies completed on rats show that fish oil makes fat cells insulin resistant and muscle cells insulin receptive. A hormone secreted by your pancreas, insulin helps your body use blood sugar by escorting it into cells. Insulin, when levels are high enough, also prevents fat release from fat cells. Therefore, when your fat cells become insulin resistant, they're less susceptible to the fat-preserving effects of the hormone. When your muscle cells become more receptive to insulin, more sugar can enter and be burned for energy. Scientists call this shift in blood sugar storage "improved nutrient partitioning." I like to call it "starving the fat, feeding the muscle," because that's precisely what happens.

Take fish oil for a day, and you won't notice much. Take it for a few weeks, and you'll notice fat shrinking and muscle growing. Researchers at the University of Western Ontario have demonstrated that in just 3 weeks of supplementing with fish oil (no exercise required), men and women can drop 2 pounds of fat and gain 2 pounds of lean mass.

In addition to boosting metabolism and helping you burn fat and build muscle, fish-oil supplements lead to the following benefits.

Reduced risk of diabetes. Diabetes is a condition marked by a dramatically reduced ability to tolerate glucose (blood sugar) and insulin. People with diabetes have chronically high insulin levels, trapping fat in the fat cells and causing an increase in fat storage. They also have chronically high blood sugar despite the increased insulin in the blood. Because fish oil makes your muscle cells more receptive to insulin and your fat cells less receptive to it, it helps better direct and control blood sugar.

Reduced risk of cardiovascular disease and stroke. Your blood vessel walls undergo structural damage all the time. It's when a few damaged areas become inflamed that different materials begin to gum up the works. Once a blood vessel wall becomes inflamed, blood cells and blood fats stick to the inflamed area. Plaque forms and narrows the blood vessel, which increases blood pressure and eventually cuts off blood flow. Fish oil reduces levels of pro-inflammatory cytokines throughout the body, making it less likely that your blood vessels will become inflamed.

Less joint pain. Like heart disease and stroke, arthritis and joint pain are also related to inflammation. When your joints become chronically inflamed, damage and pain follows. Fish oil helps keep inflammation in check, reducing the painful symptoms of arthritis.

Follow these pointers when shopping for your fish-oil supplement.

- Check the Nutrition Facts label and make sure your supplement contains a blend of EPA and DHA. A supplement that contains only one or the other won't work as effectively as one that contains both.
- Add up the amounts of EPA and DHA listed on the back of the product and make sure the total is at least 300 milligrams per capsule. Don't be confused by the numbers here. Most commercially available fish-oil supplements contain 1,000 milligrams of *fish oil* per capsule. Of that amount, your product should contain somewhere between 300 milligrams (30 percent) and 600 milligrams (60 percent) of *total EPA plus DHA*.
- When most people think of fish oil, they think of cod-liver oil. But this isn't the kind of fish oil you need. Your fish oil should come from salmon, menhaden, anchovy, sardine, or crilla. Check the list of ingredients and make sure you're buying a supplement that contains oil from one or more of these fish.
- Shop at discount warehouses like Sam's Club or Costco. These stores offer great deals on bulk fish-oil supplements. It's a good idea to have a big bottle on hand at all times since you'll be taking quite a few capsules each day—I recommend somewhere between 6 and 10 per day (1 or 2 capsules with each meal).

PROTEIN SUPPLEMENTS

When compared with carbohydrates and fat, protein emerges as the true superstar of your macronutrient metabolism-boosting team. You can, of course, consume your protein from either food or supplements. In the Metabolism Advantage plan, I recommend you do both.

Now, contrary to what protein supplement marketers would have you believe, these supplements aren't magical muscle-building, fat-burning potions. That said, they have an important role in your metabolism-boosting arsenal. They provide a really convenient way of getting a quick dose of muscle-building, metabolism-boosting amino acids when you are on the go and don't have time for a meal. For example, these powders become particularly important during and right after a workout, when you probably don't have a steak or burger stashed in your gym bag.

Use these pointers to pick the right protein powder for you.

Reach for a milk protein blend. You'll find a wide variety of protein types on the market today, including soy protein, rice protein, and milk protein extracts such as casein and whey. For everyday use—as in the Super Shakes you'll make on the 8-week program—nothing compares to a good milk protein blend. Your body digests this blend more slowly than it does other isolated protein types, increasing muscle protein synthesis and decreasing muscle protein breakdown.

These blends also provide a wider range of amino acids, a factor that also encourages muscle growth and discourages muscle break-down. In fact, when researchers Robert Demling, MD, and Leslie DeSanti, RN, of Brigham and Women's Hospital in Boston, put men on a 12-week weight-training program, those who took a milk protein blend supplement lost more fat and gained more muscle than those who took regular whey protein.

If you can't tolerate milk protein blends, use a rice protein extract. A small number of people can't tolerate milk proteins very well. Now, this isn't lactose intolerance, a condition related to milk sugar. Instead, this is intolerance to the protein itself. If you have this intolerance and take a milk protein blend, you'll either get gassy and bloated or stuffy and full of mucus. As you might imagine, neither is desirable. In this case, use a rice protein extract instead. Unlike soy protein, which is low in one of the essential amino acids, rice protein supplements have been fortified with extra amino acids, making them complete. Rice protein is also generally more easily tolerated than soy. Finally, there's enough research showing that soy protein extracts negatively affect the balance of the hormones estrogen and testosterone to make me recommend avoiding soy.

Flip the bottle and read the ingredients. Manufacturers refer to their blends by a few different aliases. The most confusing situation of all happens with milk blends. To know whether you have the right product, check the label. If the product you're holding contains any of the following as one of its first three ingredients, you're on the right track: calcium caseinate isolate or concentrate, casein isolate or concentrate, or milk protein isolate or concentrate.

No sugars, please. Make sure that your protein supplement contains mostly protein. Many of the popular protein products have a lot of sugar and fat sneaked into them in an attempt to improve flavor. Leave these on the shelves. The product you choose should contain 20 to 25 grams of protein per serving, with less than 4 grams of carbohydrate and less than 4 grams of fat per serving.

If you get up and go to the health food store, supermarket, or vitamin supplement store right now, you'll easily get frustrated because you probably won't find a protein supplement that meets all of the previously mentioned requirements. So I want to make things easy for you. I've tried most of the protein supplements on the market and really recommend only one: Metabolic Drive. Manufactured by Biotest, this product is one of the best-tasting, highest-quality protein supplements on the market today. (Consult www.MetabolismAdvantage.com for information on where to find this product.) Of course, if you find another supplement that meets all the standards I outlined, tastes great, and dissolves well in smoothies, go ahead and use it—and e-mail me through my Web site to let me know about it.

As you'll be using your protein supplements to help you get your protein power when you don't have whole food protein readily available, I don't recommend a specific amount of supplemental protein. However, if you have a couple of Super Shakes each day, you'll end up using two to four scoops of protein powder daily.

GREENS SUPPLEMENTS

In the Metabolism Advantage nutrition plan, you learned to always eat vegetables with protein. Since you'll eat protein multiple times a day—at every meal and snack—you'll also eat vegetables multiple times a day. In fact, for best results, I recommend that my clients eat 10 servings of fruits and vegetables a day, if not more.

Sounds a bit daunting, doesn't it? That's because it is. Unless you're a professional chef or currently unemployed (and therefore have a lot of time on your hands), you might not have the time to prepare vegetables that often. In fact, statistics show the following abysmal numbers.

- Less than 1 percent of men and 4 percent of women ages 18 to 24 eat five daily servings of fruits and veggies.
- Less than 6 percent of men and 9 percent of women ages 25 to 34 eat five daily servings of fruits and veggies.
- Less than 14 percent of men and 16 percent of women ages 35 to 49 eat five daily servings of fruits and veggies
- Less than 24 percent of men and 22 percent of women ages 50 to 64 eat five daily servings of fruits and veggies.

So what can you do? Look to veggie supplements to help you meet your daily vegetable goals. These "greens powders" are essentially fruits and veggies that have been compacted and distilled into powdered form. These supplements contain a variety of ingredients, including an assortment of grasses and green vegetables such as spinach and broccoli.

Although I don't recommend that you use a greens powder *instead of* eating real food, I do recommend that you take one *in conjunction with* real food. It will help fill in the dietary gaps, allowing you to meet your fruit and vegetable quota. Just one serving of this powder supplies your body with the equivalent of seven servings of fruits and vegetables.

More important, several recent research studies have shown that supplementation with greens powder can offer improvement in the following areas.

Energy and vitality. Study participants who took a greens supplement for 3 months reported higher levels of energy and vitality than other participants who took a placebo supplement. Also, participants who took the greens supplement tended to score better on mental health, overall health, and well-being scales.

Antioxidant status. After taking a greens supplement, study participants had significantly increased levels of antioxidants in their blood.

Bone health. Study participants who took greens products improved their overall bone formation, reducing their risk of the bone-thinning disease osteoporosis. The greens may work by balancing dietary acids, making it less likely that your body will leach minerals out of your bones to lower blood acid levels. Greens also contain many micronutrients needed for bone health.

Of course, if you're able to eat 10 servings of fruits and veggies every day, you probably don't need to supplement with greens powders. On the other hand, if you fall short even once in a while, you should add these to your daily plan. In the Metabolism Advantage plan, you'll use these supplements when making shakes and smoothies, so you'll typically take in 1 or 2 servings of greens supplements per day.

You'll find many different types of greens supplements on the market. As with protein supplements, they're not all created equal. Many simply taste horrific, and some, no matter the speed and power of your blender, won't dissolve in liquid. The only brand that has been studied extensively and has good, peer-reviewed research to back it up is called Greens+. (For ordering information, consult www.Metabolism Advantage.com.)

CREATINE

Way back in 1926, the *Journal of Biological Chemistry* first published a study linking creatine supplementation with increases in muscle size. Since then, more than 500 studies have evaluated the effects of creatine on muscle function. Its effectiveness and safety are now so well documented that there are few exercise physiologists who don't recommend the stuff to exercisers.

So what is creatine? It is a naturally occurring compound that is present in the food we eat, especially red meat. If you eat 8 ounces of steak, you'll get 1 gram of creatine, so you can't avoid the stuff even if you wanted to. That said, you wouldn't want to. As I just mentioned, creatine delivers some amazing benefits.

Creatine also occurs naturally in your body. That's right, your cells are already loaded with it, and for good reason. Creatine is an energy-producing molecule, necessary for everything from muscle movement to thought (the brain requires energy just as the muscles do). When you add a little extra creatine to your diet, you end up with better energy production, and that translates to more strength.

Creatine supplements work by super-hydrating your muscles, swelling and stretching the muscle cells. Researchers theorize that the lining of the muscle contains structural features that sense this swelling and respond by telling the muscle to grow larger to accommodate this good type of swelling. The upshot? Studies show that creatine supplements improve strength by 5 to 15 percent and sprint performance by 1 to 5 percent. It's so powerful that supplementation can increase muscle strength and size substantially in just 5 days, even in older adults. The supplement also boosts metabolic rate.

Yet, when most people think of creatine, they think of bulky weightlifters. That's because it has gotten a lot of attention for its ergogenic (performance-boosting) properties. Although studies repeatedly have demonstrated creatine's ability to improve athletic performance in a variety of activities, there's even more good news.

Did you know that creatine supplementation has been shown to improve memory and intelligence in vegetarians? How about that animal and human studies show that it improves and protects the nervous system in conditions such as Parkinson's disease, Huntington's disease , and amyotrophic lateral sclerosis (ALS, also known as Lou Gehrig's disease)? For example, a study at Cornell University Medical Center concluded that creatine was twice as effective as the prescription drug riluzole in extending the lives of mice with ALS.

There's still more. Research shows that creatine supplementation may reduce heart disease risk by lowering blood concentrations of homocysteine, an amino acid linked to heart disease.

Surprised? Most people are. They don't know about any of those benefits because the media has focused its attention on the athletic-performance angle. It's a shame, because the evidence is mounting that creatine may be just what the doctor ordered, especially for older people who exercise.

Now, of course, you still may have some reservations about creatine, probably because of the pesky media bombarding you with misinformation about the stuff. For example, the worst offense is the comparison some journalists (no scientist would make this mistake) make between creatine and anabolic steroids. Steroids and creatine have about as much in common as a river and a rock. They have no similar chemical characteristics, no similar characteristics in the body, no similar characteristics, period. Got that? None.

Study after study after study has shown that not only is creatine incredibly effective, it's also safe. A large review of many studies published in the *Journal of Sports Medicine and Physical Fitness* determined that creatine produces no adverse side effects with regard to gastrointestinal, cardiovascular, musculoskeletal, kidney, or liver functions. This report concluded, "The only documented side effect is an increase in [lean] body mass." Got that?

How much should you take? The Metabolism Advantage plan recommends 3 to 5 grams every day. One teaspoon contains 5 grams of creatine, so if you add ½ teaspoon to each of two daily Metabolism Advantage Super Shakes, they will be that much more super!

How do you choose which creatine to buy? Although there are a lot of fancy and expensive creatine supplements on the market today, if you find an inexpensive, powdered, basic creatine monohydrate product, you'll do fine.

POSTWORKOUT RECOVERY DRINKS

Recovery nutrition is one of the hottest current topics in the supplement world. In labs around the world, researchers are busy looking at how simple combinations of proteins and carbohydrates can improve athletic performance, body composition, and health. Studies show that protein synthesis (the process of building up muscles) is stimulated and protein breakdown (the process of tearing down muscles) is suppressed when you consume the right type of nutrients right after exercise.

What types of nutrients am I talking about here? The absolute best workout nutrition plans incorporate liquid supplements containing rapidly digested protein and carbohydrates. You don't need any fancy ingredients. You just need to down the drink at the right times—during and after your workouts. In fact, calling these recovery drinks supplements is even a bit of a stretch since most of them are just fast-digesting liquid carbohydrates in the form of sugar and protein in the form of isolated milk proteins.

When you time it right, you can expect the following benefits from your recovery drink.

BENEFIT #1: Improved recovery from exercise (including better performance in subsequent exercise sessions)

BENEFIT #2: Less muscle soreness after exercise

BENEFIT #3: Increased ability to build muscle

BENEFIT #4: Improved ability to fight off the common cold

BENEFIT #5: Improved bone mass and reduced risk of bone weakening with age

BENEFIT #6: Improved fat burning with your next exercise session, regardless of the type of exercise

With all of these benefits—more muscle, stronger bones, enhanced immunity—it should come as no surprise that all of my personal clients, from soccer players to soccer moms, are using recovery drinks.

By drinking a supplement with rapidly digested carbs and protein during and immediately after your exercise sessions, you'll take advantage of what some scientists call the exercise window of opportunity. During this window, your muscles are primed to accept nutrients that can stimulate muscle repair, muscle growth, and muscle strength. Feed your body properly while this window is open, and you'll get the benefits listed above. Skip this opportunity, and you'll suffer the consequences.

Here's one way to make sense of this window concept. Imagine that you have two windows at the front of your house. Imagine also that one window is fully open and the other is open only 25 percent of the way. If you were to throw a bucket of water at each of the windows, the window that's fully open would allow all of that water in, while the window that's only 25 percent open would let in only a small amount. This is the case with your muscles. During and after a workout, the "muscle window" is fully open. As soon as you stop exercising, however, it begins to slowly close. As each minute ticks by, the opening becomes smaller and smaller. Therefore, in order to get the best results from your exercise program, you must feed your muscles the right nutrients while the window is fully open.

A recovery drink allows you to take advantage of this postworkout window of opportunity. Unlike food, these drinks are easy to toss in your gym bag. No matter how nasty your socks, your recovery drink will stay fresh!

What type of drink should you choose? Look for a formulated recovery drink that contains rapidly digested carbohydrates (like dextrose or glucose) and proteins (like whey protein). Why am I recommending sugar (dextrose/glucose)? Isn't sugar bad? Well, by now you should know that there's no such thing as a good or bad food, only good and bad times to eat certain foods. During this one instance—during and just after your workouts—sugar offers several benefits. During the rest of the day, however, you want to avoid it.

Personally, I drink and highly recommend a recovery drink called Surge. This product is manufactured by Biotest and is probably the best-tasting, highest-quality recovery drink on the market. (Consult www.MetabolismAdvantage.com for ordering information.)

5

The Metabolism Advantage Exercise Plan

Incinerate 500 to 1,000 daily calories with these Metabolism Advantage moves

When Alex first came to me, he was carrying 180 pounds on his 5'6" frame. He had been chubby since childhood and had gained more weight during and after college.

He ran 2 miles a day and ate almost nothing, yet he couldn't get his weight to budge. At 30 percent fat, the 23-year-old was officially considered obese. I put Alex on the Metabolism Advantage exercise program you'll find in this chapter. In just 8 weeks, he dropped 19 pounds of fat and gained 12 pounds of lean mass, lowering his body fat to 20 percent. He accomplished all of this while eating 500 to 700 *additional* daily calories. Here's how Alex burned off his blubber—and how you will do the same.

- **During exercise:** The Metabolism Advantage exercise plan includes three 60-minute strength-training sessions and three

30-minute cardio sessions each week. This amount of exercise will burn roughly 300 to 600 calories per day during your workouts.

- **After exercise:** Because of the intensity of the Metabolism Advantage workouts, your body will continue to burn calories at a higher rate *after you leave the gym.* After your weight-training sessions, for example, your muscles will restock fuel and repair proteins for roughly 12 to 24 hours, elevating your metabolism by anywhere from 5 to 10 percent. Finally, research shows that intense weightlifting and cardio boosts the calories your body burns to digest food at your next meal by as much as 73 percent. All told, you can expect to burn an additional 100 to 200 calories per day due to this afterburn.

- **All day long:** Your weight-training sessions will build larger, stronger muscle fibers that must gobble up more calories to maintain themselves. All the organs in your body burn calories both to conduct their daily functions and to renew themselves. Your muscles are no exception. The more muscle you have, the faster your metabolism runs. On the Metabolism Advantage plan, you can expect to increase your resting metabolism by 7 percent or more. As long as you stick with the program, this boost is permanent, allowing you to burn up to 100 to 200 additional calories per day.

All told, the Metabolism Advantage exercise plan will boost calorie burning by 500 to 1,000 calories daily during your workouts, after your workouts, and all day long—all as a result of your exercise alone.

No matter how much you currently exercise—ranging from not at all to hours a day—the Metabolism Advantage exercise plan can take you from a sluggish metabolism to a speedy one. The program will help reverse the age-related drop in metabolism caused by either inactivity or the wrong types of activity. Indeed, you can exercise—

even exercise a lot—and still have a slow metabolism. In order to speed things up, you must do the right types and right amounts of exercise.

Metabolism-Boosting Exercise

The prevalence of bestselling diet books that promise fantastic results in just 8 or fewer minutes a day has led me to this conclusion: Many people want results, but they don't want to put in the time needed to get those results.

While I certainly would love to sell millions of books (who doesn't?), I also want you to reach your goals. So I won't sugarcoat things for you. To speed up your metabolism in a permanent way, you have to spend some serious time in the gym. According to piles and piles of well-conducted scientific studies, you must do the following in order to boost metabolism and shed fat.

Exercise for at least 5 hours a week. Research from the University of Wyoming clearly demonstrates that it takes at least 5 hours a week to see real body composition results. In this survey of more than 1,000 people, researchers concluded that people who work out for less time than that tend to be unhappy with the way they look and feel. On the other hand, people who work out for more than 5 hours a week tend to be happy with the way they look and feel. According to scientifically based U.S. government guidelines, you must exercise for 30 minutes a day to improve your health and 60 minutes a day to burn fat. In research conducted on weight gainers and maintainers, maintainers spent 80 minutes or more per day exercising, whereas gainers spent 20 minutes or less.

Because of that research and more, the Metabolism Advantage exercise plan includes six weekly workouts that add up to roughly 5 hours of exercise a week. Now, if you're doing no exercise at the moment, that may seem like a heck of a lot of time. Let's put things in perspective. When you consider that the average North American watches about 28 hours of television per week (that's right, 28), finding 5 hours to exercise shouldn't seem so problematic. Just turn off *COPS*, Spike TV's James Bond-a-thon, or the current race on Speedvision, put on your sneaks, and get to the gym!

I don't want to hear any grumbling about your demanding job or busy home life. No matter what your current schedule, you can succeed on this program. How do I know? I've seen all types of people of all ages, from 30-year-old professionals to 60-year-old empty nesters, fit these workouts into their lives. To date, I have not met a client who was too busy to make this program work. Finding time to exercise is a mindset. Do you want to lose fat, gain muscle, and boost your metabolism 24 hours a day? Then commit yourself to this program, put your workouts on the calendar, and make them nonnegotiable.

Make every workout count. To maximize your afterburn and your resting metabolic rate (RMR), you'll focus on intense strengthening and cardio workouts. In the weight room, at least once a week, you'll lift weights that are heavy enough to completely fatigue your muscles within 5 to 7 repetitions. This high-resistance, low-repetition method will target the maximum number of muscle fibers in each workout. The more muscle fibers you fatigue *during* your workout, the more your body must repair *after* your workout, maximizing your afterburn. The same is true of cardio. The Metabolism Advantage cardio plan prescribes interval training. In these high-intensity workouts, you'll alternate between surges of fast-paced cardio, which boost your heart rate above 90 percent of your maximum, and a slower recovery pace. Studies show that this type of intense cardio revs up your metabolism not only during your workout but also for many hours afterward.

Give your body time to recover. To build a faster metabolism, you must build bigger muscles. To build bigger muscles, you must apply the principles of the stress-recovery cycle. You stress your muscles during your weight-training and cardio workouts, then you rest them, giving them time to recover. During this recovery phase, your muscles restock their fuel stores, repair microtrauma, and replace protein. If you stress and stress and stress your muscles and provide no recovery time, you hinder your results and may even end up over-trained, a condition that may even *slow* your metabolism. So, no matter how gung-ho you are, resist the urge to earn extra credit by sneaking in extra workouts!

During the first 8 weeks of the main Metabolism Advantage plan, you'll take 1 day off each week, giving your body the downtime it needs to repair itself. (In subsequent weeks or in alternate plans, you may take an additional day off. See Chapters 9 and 10 for details.) Through upper-body, lower-body, and total-body sessions, you'll also strength train each major muscle group just twice a week. This provides the stimulus your muscles need to grow as well as the rest they need to repair themselves. You can alter this schedule to fit your lifestyle and goals (Chapter 9 will show you how), but you must always give your muscles the rest they need.

Change your program every 4 weeks. No matter how intense your workouts, if you do the same type of exercises week after week, your body may adapt to those exercises, and your results may plateau. As with any other stressor (exercise is a stressor, you know—a good one, but a stressor nonetheless), the body adapts to all demands placed upon it. Therefore, to prevent it from adapting too well to the program (thereby leaving you stalled out and making no further progress), the Metabolism Advantage plan changes every 4 weeks.

During weeks 1 through 4, you'll repeatedly complete three strength-training workouts: one for the upper body, one for the lower body, and one total-body session. During this time, you'll adapt to these movements. As you gain strength, you'll lift heavier weights. By week 4, however, these workouts will become as familiar to you as your morning commute. So, to maximize afterburn, you'll challenge your muscles—and mind—with a completely new set of moves. For the same reason, your cardio workouts will change as well.

EXERCISE BY THE 90 PERCENT RULE

On the Metabolism Advantage exercise plan, you need not adhere to the program 100 percent of the time. I'm putting you under no pressure to be perfect. Since the difference between 90 percent and 100 percent is negligible, I allow and encourage 10 percent "wiggle room."

So how can you best follow the 90 percent rule when it comes to exercise? Let's do the math.

For the main Metabolism Advantage exercise plan, you're going to do an average of six exercise sessions per week. That translates to about 24 exercise sessions per month. Ten percent of that is about 2.4 total workouts. Therefore, in addition to your formal day off each week, you have 2 or 3 more days off (or light days) to play with each month.

If you follow the plan 100 percent of the time, that's great. Keep it up! If you need to skip a workout every now and then, rest assured that you'll still meet your goals as long as you follow the 90 percent rule.

Be flexible. In the following pages, you'll find one way to execute the Metabolism Advantage exercise plan. I'd be oversimplifying things, however, if I told you it was the only way. As long as you follow the principles of the plan—by completing intense workouts, giving your body time to recover, and changing your program every 4 weeks—you can easily customize it to your personal goals and lifestyle and still reap the results. In fact, doing so will increase your success. When you design a program that fits your lifestyle, you increase your odds of sticking to it! In Chapter 9, you'll find everything you need to know to do just that.

Metabolism Advantage Strength Training

Whether you're young or old, strength training is critical to your metabolism and overall well-being. Even if you're in your nineties, regular strength training can triple your strength.

If you do only cardio and no strength training, you can expect to lose strength, gain fat, struggle with lower-back pain, and eventually become more reliant on others for physical tasks. Balance the right types of cardio workouts with the right type of strength training, however, and you can expect to build and preserve muscle as you age and remain lean, strong, and injury-free.

When you lift weights, you challenge your muscles to do something they are unaccustomed to doing. This damages muscle fibers, creating areas of dead and dying tissue. Your immune system then sends in specialized cells called leukocytes and macrophages to break down both the damaged tissue and some healthy tissue. Although this sounds like a bad thing, it's not. Once the leukocytes and macrophages finish their demolition duty, more immune cells rush in. These create new, thicker, stronger proteins to replace the proteins that the leukocytes and macrophages just destroyed and hauled away.

Think of your immune cells as construction workers who have been hired to repair a hurricane-ravaged house. They tear off the roof and other damaged structures and then nail on new shingles and other materials, creating a stronger house able to withstand higher-force winds. During their demolition and construction work, these workers burn a lot of calories.

It's the same with your immune cells. During the 24 hours after your workout, these busy cells elevate your metabolism by 5 to 10 percent. The bigger you are, the more muscle you damage during a workout, giving you an even greater afterburn.

These bigger, stronger muscle fibers increase your metabolism 24 hours a day. All tissues in your body—including your muscles—go through a regular program of turnover. You may be familiar with skin turnover, for example. Every day, old skin flakes off and new skin forms underneath. Every organ in your body goes through this process, which gobbles up a great number of calories. You can't do much to speed up the turnover rates of most of your organs, but you *can* increase the turnover rate of your muscles. The more muscle you have, the more muscle cells your body must continually recycle. As I've mentioned, 1 extra pound of muscle burns up to 50 extra calories a day. Add 5 pounds of tight, lean muscle, and you'll boost your body's energy needs by 250 calories per day.

For optimal results, you'll do the following on the Metabolism Advantage plan.

Mix high-intensity with moderate-intensity lifting. You've probably heard at least three theories about how much weight and how many repetitions you should complete when weightlifting. Guys who are after big muscle will tell you to do heavy weights and low reps. Some exercise physiologists recommend the standard 10 to 12 reps. And some personal trainers tell women to do 15 or more reps to tone rather than bulk. Who's right? As it turns out, no one.

To boost your metabolism to the max, you need to perform a combination of high-intensity, low-repetition training and moderate-intensity, moderate-weight training. This varied approach will ensure that you target all of your muscle fibers, boosting your afterburn and overall metabolism.

Typical strength-training plans that tell you to lift a weight 8, 10, or 15 times target predominantly type I and IIa fibers. When you weight train, these fibers attempt to shoulder the load. Type IIb fibers, a third type, are difficult to target, but seeking them out is well worth the effort. If you work only your type I and type IIa fibers, you leave roughly a third of your muscle fibers untrained. This reduces your burn during and after your workout and prevents you from maximizing your RMR.

To work and break down type IIb fibers, you need to lift a weight that's heavy enough to fatigue the muscle you are working in 5 to 7 reps. (Some programs targeting IIb fibers recommend working in the 1-to-3-rep range as well.) That's why, during two of your weekly weight workouts on the main Metabolism Advantage program, you'll try to reach muscle failure within 5 to 7 repetitions. In other words, you will choose a weight that you can lift no more than seven times. If you tried to bang out another rep, you wouldn't be able to lift the bar. This type of weightlifting will help to target all of your muscle fibers.

So if low-rep, high-intensity lifting trains all of your muscle fibers, why not lift this way all the time? This type of lifting is very stressful to your nervous system. Do it more than twice a week, and you raise your risk of burnout and injury to joints and other supporting structures. Also, mixing up your weights and reps provides variety in your program, which helps stimulate muscle growth. That's why one of your weekly workouts calls for 8 to 10 reps rather than 5 to 7. It's also why the various weightlifting programs you'll find in Chapter 9 include a variety of reps.

Do compound movements instead of isolation movements. Roughly 80 percent of the weightlifting moves you'll find in the pages that follow consist of compound movements. In contrast to isolation exercises, such as preacher curls that zero in on the biceps muscles, compound movements target more than one muscle at a time by working more than one joint at a time. This increases your calorie burn during your workout because you're using more muscles at once. It also makes each workout more efficient.

There are various types of compound-movement exercises. Some of them, such as the bench press, require multiple muscles to complete one movement. To press the bar away from your chest, you must use your deltoids (shoulders), pectorals (chest), lats (back), triceps (upper arms), and rotator cuff (small muscles around the shoulder joint). Other exercises work the entire body in multiple movements. For example, in the push press, you work your legs as you squat, your core as you extend to standing, and your shoulders as you hoist the bar overhead. Finally, for some of the exercises, you'll use a Swiss ball to put you off-balance. This forces you to work your core—and many other muscles—to remain balanced.

Use a balanced approach. When left to their own devices, most people do the exercises they like and avoid the ones they hate. The result: They make their already strong muscles stronger and their weaker muscles even weaker! The Metabolism Advantage plan will help you work all of the muscle groups in your body equally. In addition to helping to build muscle throughout your body—creating more overall muscle and boosting your metabolism—this balanced approach helps prevent injuries due to muscle imbalances. It also improves your posture. And hey, it creates a more symmetrical appearance.

Recover after every set. On the main Metabolism Advantage program, your muscles will need roughly 1 to 1½ minutes to rest between sets. (In Chapter 9, you'll find additional routines that call for a different recovery time.)

Lift fast. To recruit the maximum number of muscle fibers, lift as quickly as you can, but lower the weight fairly slowly, to a count of three. Because you'll lift heavy weights, *fast* is obviously a relative term here, so just put everything you have behind each lift. I want you to focus all of your mental energy on the lift, not on counting, so work with a partner to egg you on during the lifting phase of the movement and encourage you to slow things down during the lowering phase.

The Workouts

In the following pages, you'll find two lower-body, two upper-body, and two total-body strength-training workouts. To find the right weight for you, take a list of all of the exercises in the program to the gym and, exercise by exercise, experiment with different weights until you find the right weight to fatigue your muscles in either 5 reps (for the upper- and lower-body workouts) or 8 reps (for the total-body workout). This means, seriously, that if someone held a gun to your head, you couldn't do another rep beyond the 5 or 8 that you just completed—not even to save your life.

Warm up before each workout with 5 minutes of light cardio and cool down afterward with another 5 minutes of light cardio.

Lower Body

■ BARBELL SQUAT
Quads, Glutes, Hamstrings

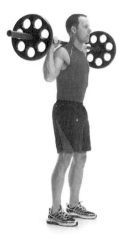 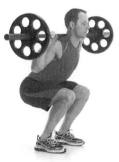

A Position a barbell along the backs of your shoulders, holding the bar with an overhand grip.

B With your body weight equally distributed between your heels and forefeet, bend your knees, lowering your torso until your thighs are parallel to the floor. Keep your head forward, your back straight, and your feet flat on the floor.

Extend your knees and hips and rise until your legs are straight. Complete 2 sets of 5 to 7 reps.

■ OVERHEAD BARBELL SQUAT

Quads, Core Muscles

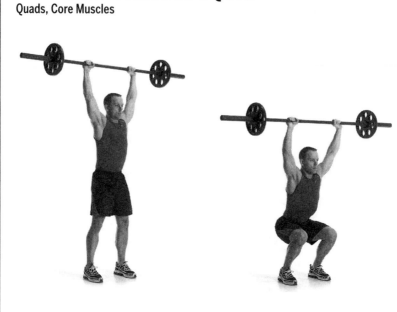

A Stand holding a barbell overhead, with your arms extended.

B With your body weight equally distributed between your heels and forefeet, bend your knees, lowering your torso until your thighs are parallel to the floor. Keep your head forward, your back straight, and your feet flat on the floor.

Extend your knees and hips and rise until your legs are straight. Complete 2 sets of 5 to 7 reps.

■ BARBELL DEADLIFT
Glutes, Hamstrings, Lower Back

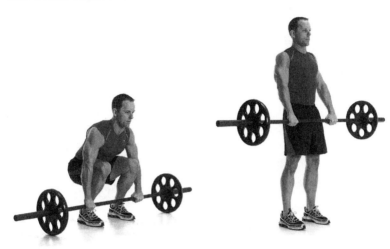

A Place a barbell on the floor and stand with your feet hip-width apart under the center of the bar. Bend your knees, squat down, and grasp the bar with an overhand grip, with your hands shoulder-width or slightly farther apart.

B Keeping your arms and back straight, extend your knees and hips as you lift the bar and stand. As you lift, keep the bar close to your body. Pull your shoulders back at the top of the lift. Complete 3 sets of 5 to 7 reps.

DUMBBELL WALKING LUNGE

Glutes, Hamstrings, Quads

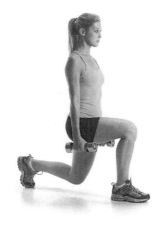 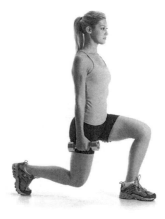

A Hold a pair of dumbbells at your sides. Lunge forward with your right leg, landing on your heel and then your forefoot. Lower your body by bending your knees until they both form right angles and the knee of your left leg is almost in contact with the floor.

B Step forward with your left leg, landing on your heel and then your forefoot.

Continue lunging forward until you've completed 5 to 7 repetitions on each side. Complete 2 sets.

■ SINGLE-LEG SWISS BALL LEG CURL

Hamstrings, Glutes

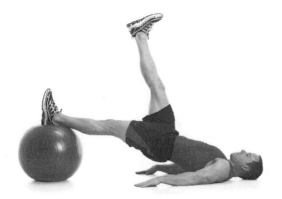

A Lie on your back with your heels and lower calves on a Swiss ball. Lift your hips until your body forms an incline. Lift your right leg into the air, balancing your body weight with just your left leg against the ball.

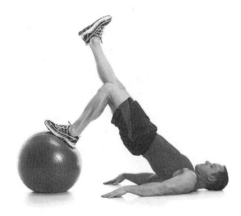

B Bend your left knee and pull the ball toward you.

Pause for a second, then slowly reverse the sequence. Complete 5 to 7 reps, then repeat with the other leg. Complete 2 sets per leg.

■ STEPUP
Glutes, Quads, Hamstrings

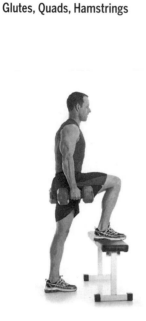
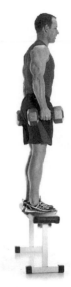

A Holding dumbbells at your sides, stand in front of a weight bench or step that's at least 12 inches high. Place your right foot on top of the bench or step.

B Press into your right foot and extend your right leg as you lift your body over the bench or step. Place your left foot on the bench or step.

Then step down onto the floor with your right foot. Keeping your torso upright, continue alternating sides until you've stepped up 5 to 7 times on each side. Complete 2 sets.

Upper Body

■ BENT-OVER BARBELL ROW
Upper and Lower Back, Biceps

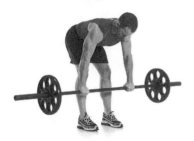 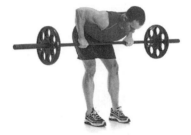

A Bend your knees slightly and bend forward with your back straight. Grasp a barbell with an overhand grip, with your hands slightly more than shoulder-width apart.

B Bend your elbows, bringing them toward the ceiling as you pull the bar toward your midsection.

Then extend your arms to the starting position, allowing your shoulders to stretch forward slightly. Complete 2 sets of 5 to 7 reps.

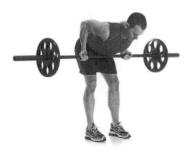

C Next, change your hand position so your palms are facing upward in an underhand grip and complete 1 more set of 5 to 7 reps.

FLAT BARBELL BENCH PRESS

Chest, Shoulders, Triceps

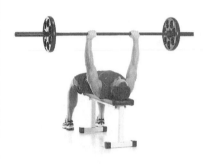 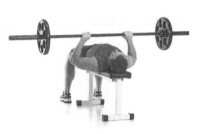

A Lie on a flat bench and position your body so the barbell on the supports is above your face. Grasp the bar with your hands shoulder-width apart. Keep your feet flat on the floor as you lift the weight off the supports and hold the bar above your chest.

B Bend your elbows to the sides as you lower the bar toward your upper chest, stopping when your elbows are in line with your torso. Pause at the bottom for a second, then press back up. Complete 5 to 7 reps.

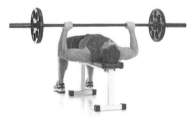 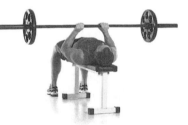

C After 1 set, change your hand position to a wide grip—more than shoulder-width apart—and complete 1 more set of 5 to 7 reps.

D Next, do the press with a narrow grip—less than shoulder-width apart—and complete 1 more set of 5 to 7 reps.

PULLUP

Upper Back, Biceps, Brachialis

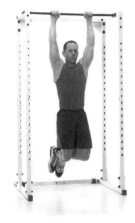

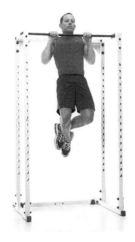

A Hang from an overhead bar with an overhand grip, with your hands shoulder-width apart.

B Pull yourself up until your chin clears the bar.

Lower and repeat, completing 5 to 7 reps.

NOTE: If you can't pull up your entire body weight, do assisted pullups, either with a partner pushing against your lower back or on a pullup machine that supports some—but not all—of your body weight.

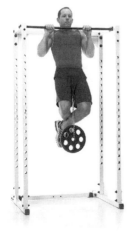

C If you can easily do 5 to 7 reps, either wear a weighted belt or hold a dumbbell between your ankles. Complete 2 sets.

■ BARBELL OVERHEAD PRESS

Shoulders, Trapezius, Triceps

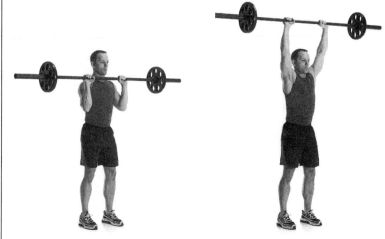

A Take a barbell off the supports of a squat rack and hold it at collarbone level with an overhand grip, with your hands shoulder-width apart.

B Walk back a step or two and then, with your knees slightly bent, press the bar overhead until your arms are straight. Lower the bar to chin level and repeat. Complete 2 sets of 5 to 7 reps.

SINGLE-ARM BARBELL BICEPS CURL

Biceps

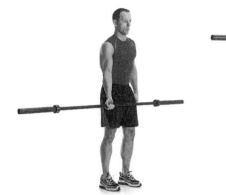 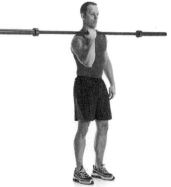

A Grasp either a long or short barbell (depending on your strength) with your right hand, holding the center of the bar in an underhand grip.

B Keeping your right elbow close to your side, raise the bar until your right forearm is vertical. Then lower it until your arm is fully extended. Complete 5 to 7 reps, then repeat with your left arm. Complete 2 sets for each arm.

■ DIP

Triceps, Chest

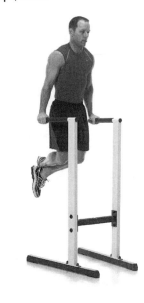
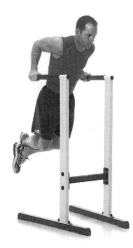

A Depending on your strength, you can do this exercise either on a dip bar with or without weight or on a dip/pullup machine that supports some of your weight. If you need added weight, either use a weighted belt or hold a dumbbell between your ankles.

Mount the dip bar or machine with your palms facing in and your arms extended.

B Keeping your elbows close to your body, bend your elbows and lower your torso until your shoulders are slightly stretched. Extend your arms and return to the starting position. Complete 2 sets of 5 to 7 reps.

Total Body

■ PUSHUP ON SWISS BALL
Chest

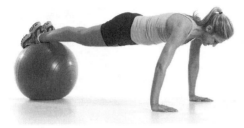

A Kneel with your belly on a Swiss ball. Roll forward until you are in a plank position, with your hands on the floor under your chest and your feet on the ball.

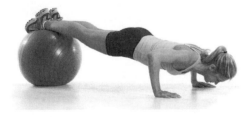

B Keeping your back straight, bend your elbows and lower your chest to the floor. Extend your arms to return to the starting position. Complete 2 sets of 8 to 10 reps.

■ SUITCASE DEADLIFT

Glutes, Hamstrings, Quads, Core Muscles

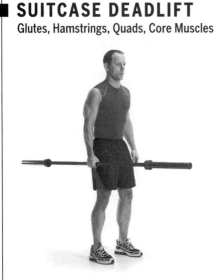 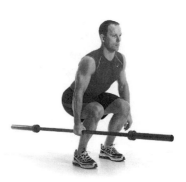

A Grasp a barbell in the center with your right hand and hold it at your right side as if it were a heavy suitcase.

B Bend your knees and squat down as if you were trying to place your suitcase on the floor. Keeping your arms and back straight, extend your knees and hips and return to the starting position. Complete 3 sets of 8 to 10 reps with each arm.

BARBELL CLEAN

Hips, Shoulders, Legs, Upper Back

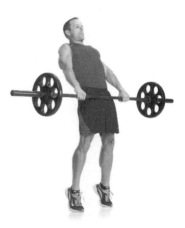

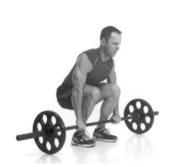

A Place a barbell on the floor and stand with your feet slightly more than hip-width apart just under the bar. Squat down and grasp the bar with an overhand grip, with your hands slightly more than shoulder-width apart. With your back arched slightly, position your shoulders over the bar.

B Extend your knees and hips as you lift the bar, at first keeping your arms extended.

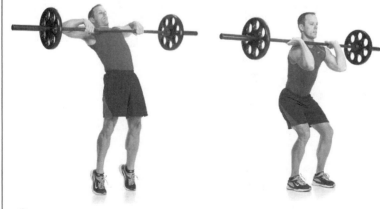

C Once the bar reaches your knees, vigorously raise your shoulders and pull the barbell up as you flex your elbows to the sides in an upright rowing motion. Keep the bar close to your body the entire time, then catch it at the top position. Lower and repeat. Complete 3 sets of 8 to 10 reps.

■ DUMBBELL OVERHEAD WALKING LUNGE

Glutes, Quads, Hamstrings, Core Muscles

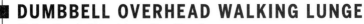

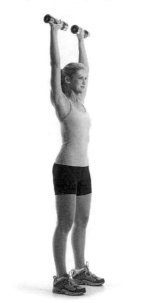
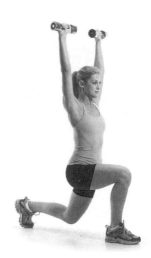

A Holding a dumbbell in each hand, stand with your arms extended overhead.

B Lunge forward with your right leg, landing on your heel and then your forefoot. Lower your body by bending your knees until they both form right angles and the knee of your left leg is almost in contact with the floor.

Then step forward with your left leg, landing on your heel and then your forefoot. Continue lunging forward until you've completed 8 to 10 repetitions on each side. Complete 2 sets.

■ BRIDGE
Core Muscles

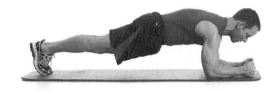

Assume a pushup position, but instead of straightening your arms, rest your weight on your forearms. Suck in your belly button and contract your glutes to flatten the arch in your lower back. Hold for 30 seconds. Complete 2 sets.

■ SIDE BRIDGE
Obliques, Abdominals

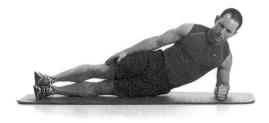

A Lie on your right side with your right forearm lined upright beneath your shoulder, perpendicular to your torso.

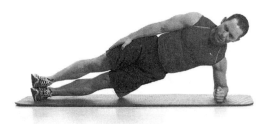

B Keeping your body straight, contract your abdominals and obliques as you raise your lower torso, hips, and legs off the floor. In the top position, your body should form a diagonal line from your feet to your head. Hold for 30 seconds.

Then switch sides and repeat. Complete 2 sets for each side.

Lower Body

■ BARBELL GOOD MORNING
Hamstrings, Lower Back

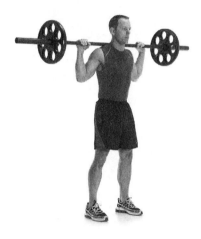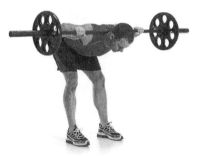

A Position a barbell along the backs of your shoulders, grasping it with an underhand grip, with your hands slightly more than shoulder-width apart.

B Bend forward from the hips as if you were bowing, but keep your back flat (not rounded). Stop when your torso is parallel to the floor.

Keeping your back and knees extended, return to the starting position. Complete 3 sets of 5 to 7 reps.

■ BARBELL HACK SQUAT

Quads, Glutes, Hamstrings

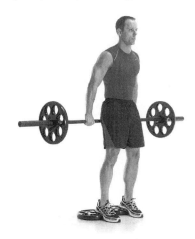
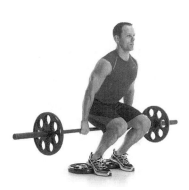

A Set a 25-pound weight plate about a foot behind each support of a squat rack. Set a barbell on the rack at about hip level and stand with your back to it, then grasp it behind your back with a shoulder-width, overhand grip. Next, slowly walk backward toward the weight plates until both your heels are elevated on them.

B Keeping your back as straight as possible, bend your knees and squat down as far as you can.

When you've reached your lowest point, push your feet into the floor to rise to the starting position. Complete 3 sets of 5 to 7 reps.

STIFF-LEG DEADLIFT
Upper and Lower Back, Glutes, Hamstrings

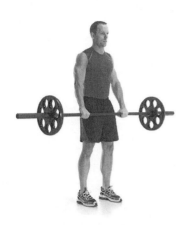

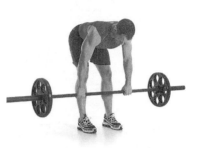

A Stand with your feet shoulder-width apart. Hold a barbell at thigh level in an overhand grip, with your hands shoulder-width apart and arms extended.

B With your knees slightly bent, bend forward from the hips, lowering the bar toward your feet until you feel a mild stretch in your hamstrings.

Then, with your knees bent, lift the bar as you stand upright. Complete 2 sets of 5 to 7 reps.

OVERHEAD DUMBBELL SQUAT

Quads, Glutes, Core Muscles

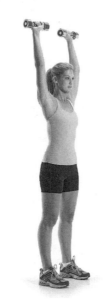 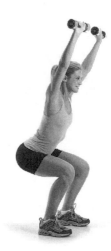

A Grasp a dumbbell in each hand and extend your arms overhead.

B Bend your knees and lower your torso until your thighs are parallel to the floor.

Then extend your knees and hips and stand up. Keep your head forward, your back straight, and your chest high. Complete 2 sets of 5 to 7 reps.

■ LEG PRESS
Quads

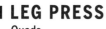

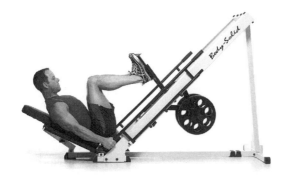

A Sit on a leg press machine with your back against the padded support. Place your feet on the platform and grasp the handles at your sides for support.

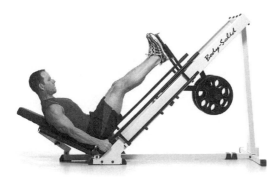

B Extend your knees and hips to push the platform away from you.

Bend your knees to return to the starting position. Keep your knees pointed up; don't let them splay outward. Also, don't let your heels rise off the platform. Complete 2 sets of 5 to 7 reps.

Upper Body

■ CHINUP
Upper Back, Biceps

You can do chinups wearing a weighted belt or with a dumbbell between your feet, assisted by a partner, or on a chinup machine.

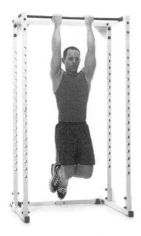 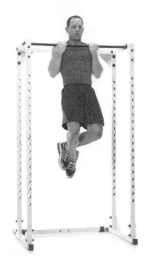

A To do a basic chinup, hang from an overhead bar with an underhand grip, with your hands shoulder-width apart.

B Extend your chest and pull yourself up until your chin clears the bar or your chest touches it.

Lower and repeat. You can do chinups with a number of different grips and hand positions. For this workout, do the following.

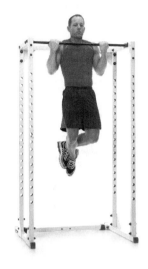

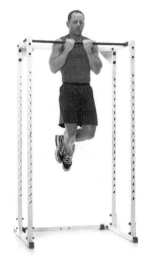

C One set of 5 to 7 reps with your hands in an overhand grip (that is, do a pullup as on page 107, with a wide grip) slightly more than shoulder-width apart.

D One set of 5 to 7 reps with your hands slightly less than shoulder-width apart.

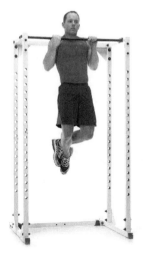

E One set of 5 to 7 reps with your right hand in an overhand grip and your left in an underhand grip. Space your hands slightly more than shoulder-width apart.

One set of 5 to 7 reps with your left hand in an overhand grip and your right in an underhand grip. Space your hands slightly more than shoulder-width apart.

The Metabolism Advantage Exercise Plan 123

■ ALTERNATING DUMBBELL INCLINE PRESS
Pectorals, Deltoids, Triceps

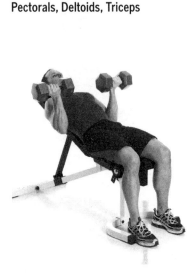 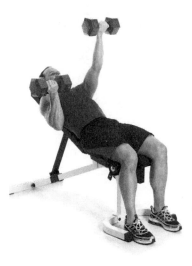

A Sit on an incline bench holding dumbbells in an underhand grip so they rest on your lower thighs. Bring the weights up to your shoulders and lean back against the bench. Position the dumbbells at the sides of your upper chest, with your elbows below the dumbbells.

B Press one dumbbell up until your arm is extended.

Lower the weight to your upper chest and repeat with the other arm. Continue alternating arms until you've completed 1 set of 5 to 7 reps.

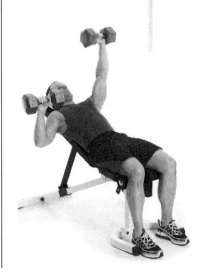

C Switch to an overhand grip and do 2 sets of 5 to 7 reps.

BARBELL CLEAN
Hips, Shoulders, Legs, Upper Back

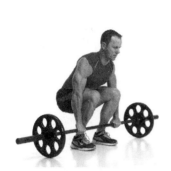

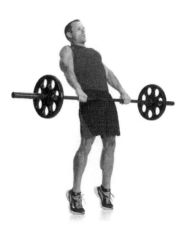

A Place a barbell on the floor and stand with your feet slightly more than hip-width apart just under the bar. Squat down and grasp the bar with an overhand grip, with your hands slightly more than shoulder width apart. With your back arched slightly, position your shoulders over the bar.

B Extend your knees and hips as you lift the bar, at first keeping your arms extended.

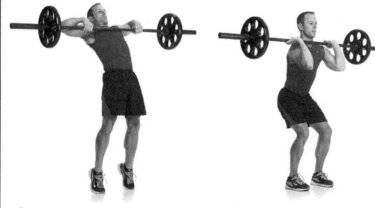

C Once the bar reaches your knees, vigorously raise your shoulders and pull the barbell up as you flex your elbows out to the sides in an upright rowing motion. Keep the bar close to your body the entire time, then catch it at the top position. Lower and repeat. Complete 2 sets of 5 to 7 reps.

ALTERNATING DUMBBELL SHOULDER PRESS ON SWISS BALL

Deltoids, Triceps

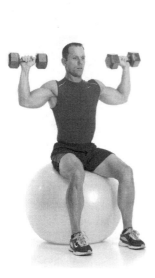 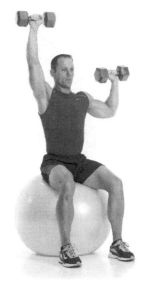

A Sit on a Swiss ball with your knees bent and your feet flat on the floor. Hold a dumbbell with an overhand grip next to each shoulder, with your elbows under your wrists.

B Press one dumbbell up until that arm is extended overhead.

Lower and repeat with the other arm. Complete 2 sets of 5 to 7 reps with each arm.

ALTERNATING DUMBBELL CURL ON SWISS BALL

Biceps

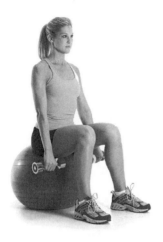
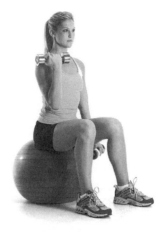

A Sit on a Swiss ball with your knees bent and your feet flat on the floor. Hold a dumbbell in an overhand grip at each side, with your arms straight.

B Keeping your elbows close to your sides, raise one dumbbell, rotating your forearm until it is vertical and your palm faces your shoulder.

Lower to the starting position and repeat with the other arm. Continue alternating left and right until you've completed 2 sets of 5 to 7 reps with each arm.

CLOSE-GRIP BENCH PRESS

Chest, Shoulders, Triceps

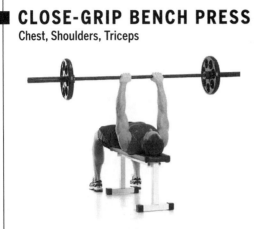

A Lie on a flat bench and position your body so the barbell on the supports is above your face. Grasp the bar with your hands less than shoulder-width apart. Keep your feet flat on the floor as you lift the weight off the supports and hold the bar above your chest.

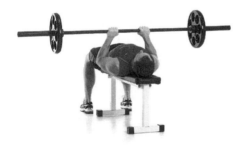

B Bend your elbows to the sides as you lower the bar toward your upper chest, stopping when your elbows are in line with your torso.

Pause at the bottom for a second, then press back up. Complete 2 sets of 5 to 7 reps.

Total Body

■ SUITCASE DEADLIFT
Glutes, Hamstrings, Quads, Core Muscles

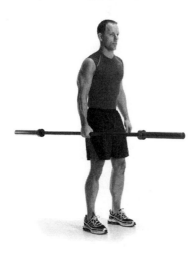
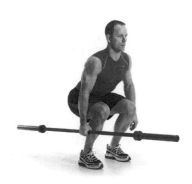

A Grasp the center of a barbell with your right hand and hold it at your right side as if it were a heavy suitcase.

B Bend your knees and squat down as if you were trying to place your suitcase on the floor.

Keeping your arms and back straight, extend your knees and hips and return to the starting position. Complete 3 sets of 8 to 10 reps with each arm.

DUMBBELL OVERHEAD WALKING LUNGE

Glutes, Quads, Hamstrings, Core Muscles

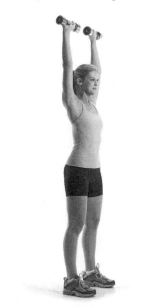 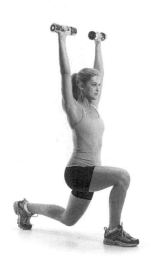

A Grasp a dumbbell in each hand and extend your arms overhead.

B Lunge forward with your right leg, landing on your heel and then your forefoot. Lower your body by bending your knees until they both form right angles and the knee of your left leg is almost in contact with the floor.

Step forward with your left leg, landing on your heel and then your forefoot. Continue lunging forward until you've completed 8 to 10 repetitions on each side. Complete 3 sets.

PUSH PRESS
Quads, Deltoids, Triceps

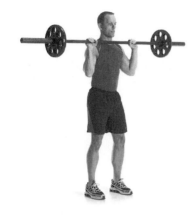

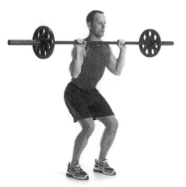

A Grasp a barbell at chest level with an overhand grip, with your hands slightly more than shoulder-width apart.

B Bend your knees and squat down.

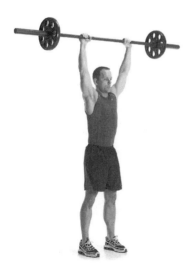

C Explosively straighten your legs as you drive the barbell up, vigorously extending your arms overhead in a shoulder press motion.

Lower the barbell to your chest and repeat. Complete 3 sets of 8 to 10 reps.

■ BENT-OVER BARBELL ROW

Upper and Lower Back, Biceps

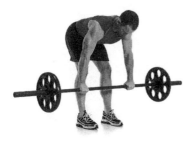 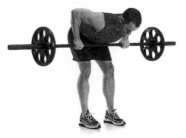

A Bend your knees slightly and bend forward with your back straight. Grasp a barbell with an overhand grip, with your hands slightly more than shoulder-width apart.

B Bend your elbows, bringing them toward the ceiling as you pull the bar toward your midsection.

Extend your arms to the starting position, allowing your shoulders to stretch forward slightly. Complete 3 sets of 8 to 10 reps.

■ BRIDGE
Core Muscles

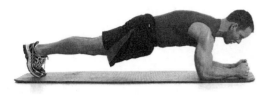

Assume a pushup position, but instead of straightening your arms, rest your weight on your forearms. Suck in your belly button and contract your glutes to flatten the arch in your lower back. Hold for 30 seconds. Complete 2 sets.

■ SIDE BRIDGE

Obliques, Abdominals

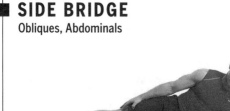

A Lie on your left side with your left forearm lined upright beneath your shoulder, perpendicular to your torso.

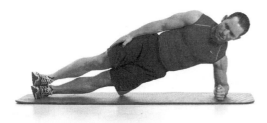

B Keeping your body straight, contract your abdominals and obliques as you raise your lower torso, hips, and legs off the floor. In the top position, your body should form a diagonal line from your feet to your head. Hold for 30 seconds.

Then switch sides and repeat. Complete 2 sets.

Metabolism Advantage Cardio

Although high-intensity cardiovascular exercise won't give you the same long-term metabolic boost as weight training, it will help you burn more calories in two ways.

1. During your workouts
2. During the 24-hour recovery window after your workouts

The biggest mistake people make? Not pushing themselves hard enough. Forget about that fat-burning zone you may have heard about. According to that theory, your body burns more fat than carbohydrate at low intensities. This is true, but your goal is to burn calories, and during your workout, it doesn't matter where those calories come from. Your muscles stock a type of fuel called glycogen (a type of stored carbohydrate) for ready access during exercise. After a workout, your muscles replace the glycogen they burned during exercise. To enable this process, the body shuts off carbohydrate burning, shuttling dietary carbohydrate to your muscles, where it's converted to glycogen. Your body still needs fuel for energy, so it switches to burning fat. So don't worry about the type of fuel you're burning during your workout. Just burn it!

High-intensity workouts burn more calories during and after exercise than low-intensity workouts. When you run, swim, bike, and do other types of high-intensity cardio, you fatigue and slightly damage your muscles, which must repair and strengthen themselves for subsequent efforts. During this recovery period, your body clears acid and metabolic byproducts from your muscles and replenishes the ATP (adenosine triphosphate, the energy source your muscles use for short bursts of power) and glycogen you burned during exercise. It also changes the makeup of protein in your muscles, replacing damaged muscle protein with new proteins capable of withstanding high-intensity endurance efforts. This process elevates your metabolism slightly for 24 to 48 hours.

How long you maintain your afterburn depends on the intensity of your effort. In one experiment, eight women cycled at either a fairly easy pace or at an extremely intense pace. When they cycled intensely, they not only burned significantly more calories during the 60-minute cycling session but also continued to burn more calories for 24 hours afterward, a metabolism boost equivalent to 150 calories.

In addition to boosting your metabolism, this type of exercise will also extend your life. The Harvard Alumni Health Study, a 4-year study of more than 17,000 men, found that only vigorous—not moderate—exercise reduced risk of death.

On the Metabolism Advantage cardio plan, you'll complete bursts of intense exercise called intervals. By pushing your pace for a specified period of time and then backing off and recovering, you'll be able to boost your VO_2 max. This is a scientific term for the maximal (max) volume (V) of oxygen (O_2) that one can consume during maximal exercise. It's a measure of your aerobic fitness.

SCIENCE MADE SIMPLE

VO_2 MAX: This scientific term stands for the maximal (max) volume (V) of oxygen (O_2) that one can consume during maximal exercise and is a measure of aerobic fitness

To perform this type of interval exercise, select two intensities and alternate between them for the prescribed number of repetitions. On a scale of 0 to 10—with 0 being comatose and 10 being the hardest you could ever work—you should hit an intensity of 9 during your 30-second intervals, 8 during 60-second intervals, and 7 during 90-second intervals. During your recovery period, aim for an intensity of 3.

Experiment to find the right high and low intensities for you. You'll know you've found the right level when you can keep the high- and low-intensity levels constant throughout the duration of the interval session. If you can't do this without excessive fatigue, you need to lower the intensity. You want to feel exhausted by the last few reps, but no sooner.

For example, during a cycling session on a stationary bike, you might cycle for 30 seconds at the bike's preset level 10 and 120 rpm, then decrease your intensity to level 1 and 80 rpm for 90 seconds. For a running interval session on a treadmill, you might run at 12 miles per hour on an incline of 5 percent for 60 seconds and walk for the next 60 seconds at 4 miles per hour on an incline of 0 percent. For rowing intervals, you might row at 40 strokes per minute for 90 seconds of high-intensity rowing, then at 20 strokes per minute for 180 seconds of low-intensity rowing.

Those are just examples of exercise modes and intensity settings. The Metabolism Advantage program doesn't lock you into only these types of exercise. That's right, you can pick whatever type of exercise you like, whether it's cycling, running, rowing, stairclimbing, swimming, or something else. As long as you follow the prescribed intensities and durations, you'll get the benefits you're looking for.

YOUR INTERVAL WORKOUTS

Here are the interval workouts you'll follow. Choose your favorite form of cardio—such as running, rowing, or cycling—to complete these workouts.

WORKOUT #1
    5-minute low-intensity cardio warmup
    Intervals: 30 seconds at high intensity, 90 seconds at low intensity
    Weeks 1–4: Perform 7 total intervals
    Weeks 5–8: Perform 10 total intervals
    5-minute low-intensity cardio cooldown

WORKOUT #2
    5-minute low-intensity cardio warmup
    Intervals: 60 seconds at high intensity, 60 seconds at low intensity
    Weeks 1–4: Perform 7 total intervals
    Weeks 5–8: Perform 10 total intervals
    5-minute low-intensity cooldown

WORKOUT #3

    5-minute low-intensity cardio warmup

    Intervals: 90 seconds at high intensity, 180 seconds at
       low intensity

    Weeks 1–4: Perform 4 total intervals

    Weeks 5–8: Perform 5 total intervals

    5-minute low-intensity cooldown

Your Weekly Schedule

In Chapter 8, you'll find 8 weeks of cardio and strength-training workouts, along with menus, self-monitoring tips, and more. This planner will help you time your meals with your workouts and balance your stress cycle with your recovery cycle. It will also help you to keep track of it all.

During each week of this planner, your exercise schedule works like this:

MONDAY: Lower-body strengthening workout
TUESDAY: Interval workout #1
WEDNESDAY: Upper-body strengthening workout
THURSDAY: Interval workout #2
FRIDAY: Total-body strengthening workout
SATURDAY: Interval workout #3
SUNDAY: Off

Keep in mind that you are not locked into this schedule. The schedule listed in Chapter 8 is an option. It's one way to do it, but it's not the only way. You can rearrange the workouts to accommodate your life—just be sure that you get them all in each week! Consult Chapter 9 for ways to modify the program to fit your lifestyle.

PART 3

THE METABOLISM ADVANTAGE PROGRAM

$$\boxed{6}$$

Your Metabolism Advantage Homework

The tools you need to make effective, lasting change

It's one thing to know what to eat, which supplements to take, and how to exercise. It's quite another to actually do all of that—over the long term.

If you've tried—and failed—to establish long-term, healthful habits many times before, then you know all too well what I'm talking about. Even though the Metabolism Advantage plan is based on effective, convenient, and achievable lifestyle changes, they are changes nonetheless. Change—whether it comes in the form of a job promotion, a new home, or new healthful habits—can feel stressful. That's why I'm assigning this bit of homework before you officially embark on your Metabolism Advantage journey. It will help you get a strong start and remain on the Metabolism Advantage plan for life.

I'd like to start your homework assignment by asking you to listen to a little story about my favorite cyclist, Lance Armstrong. Why is he my favorite? Well, partly because he's now probably the greatest cyclist of all time, and partly because in the early 1990s, he wasn't even a contender. You see, at that time, Lance was a good professional cyclist, competing and placing reasonably well yet never emerging as a dominant force in the sport. Based on this history of performance, it was clear that Lance wasn't a serious candidate for overall victory in the world's biggest cycling event, the Tour de France.

Then Lance got cancer.

After battling back from almost certain death, Lance changed. Now, seven Tour de France victories later, he has cemented his place among the greatest cyclists in history. In his book *It's Not About the Bike*, he explains why he was able to go from being an above-average professional cyclist to perhaps the greatest the sport has ever seen: "If you ever get a second chance in life for something, you've got to go all the way."

By his own admission, Lance realized that his sport is about something more than the carbohydrate drinks, the hours spent on the bike, and the tights. It's about perseverance in the midst of unknowns. As Lance notes in his book, the Tour de France "poses every conceivable element to the rider, and more: cold, heat, mountains, plains, ruts, flat tires, high winds, unspeakably bad luck, unthinkable beauty, yawning senselessness, and, above all, a great, deep self-questioning."

In my humble opinion, amid the many unknowns faced and the many lessons learned, this one lesson emerges as one of the most important. Lance overcomes cancer and Lance wins Tours because he has learned how to adapt. He practices for and adapts to varied conditions rather than letting them become setbacks. It's raining? No problem; he's ridden this course before in the rain. Heck, he's probably even ridden it in snow. The other riders see the rain as a huge disadvantage; not Lance. He owns both the sunshine and the rain.

So why am I going on and on about Lance? Because you and I can learn from his success. Even if you never, ever in a million years wish to cycle more than 100 miles a day over some of the steepest, highest-altitude mountains in the world, you can still learn from Lance. His story can help you advance your career, improve your family life, and, yes, even change your nutrition and exercise habits in order to speed up your metabolism.

You see, in order to successfully change, you must prepare for that change. That's what this chapter is all about: preparation and adaptation. Sure, you may not be battling cancer or entering the Tour de France, but you *are* in a contest, and the prize is a faster metabolism. So listen up. To change your body, fight off disease, and battle the erosion caused by Father Time, you're going to have to get prepared.

Even if you know what to eat, if the good foods aren't around when you're hungry, you're going to eat the jelly doughnut sitting on the table in the break room, right? So you need a plan, and you need to realize that sometimes it's not about the food, the exercise, or the supplements. Sometimes it's about things altogether unrelated to carbs, proteins, and fats. Rather, it's about dedication, desire, and preparation.

It's Not about the Food

Here's an example to demonstrate my point. Let's pretend that I, along with the mad scientists at the Metabolism Advantage laboratory, came up with the perfect diet for all human beings, one that solved all the ills of the world. On this diet, everyone lost weight, felt great, and doubled their life span. Heck, it made everyone feel so good that divorce and murder rates plummeted. It was the diet to end all diets. We published this diet on the good old Internet so every man, woman, and child could reap its benefits.

If this scenario were true, you know what 99 percent of the humans on the planet would do? They'd keep eating Twinkies (which, I suspect, probably wouldn't be a component of this perfect diet).

Don't believe me? Think about this. How often have you seen people who have been diagnosed with heart disease or cancer fail to take the necessary steps to improve their lifestyles? I'm sure you've seen guys with lung cancer puffing on cigarettes and guys with oxygen tubes in their noses downing fries and cheese curls. They say they *want* to change. They see doctors and nutritionists who tell them *how* to change. Yet they end up feeling guilty for *not changing*.

Why is it so hard for them to make the change? Well, unless they really don't want to change, the two biggest impediments to their success are:

1. **Their habits.** Their ingrained day-to-day diets and activities remain poor because they don't have a conscious, logical plan for changing them. As Steven Covey wrote in his book *The 7 Habits of Highly Effective People*, "we will define a habit as the intersection of knowledge, skill, and desire." Think of knowledge as the *what to do*, desire as the *want to do*, and skill as the *how to do*. If you really want to change (desire), and you learn from the lessons in this book (knowledge), and you apply those lessons (skill), you'll change your habits.

2. **They aren't ready for the tough times.** In many cases, even folks who want to change, know what to change, and start to apply the skills needed to change can get derailed. Often, just as things are getting better, the tough times, the distractions, and the negative pressures all hit. People get busy. Eating well becomes inconvenient. No one else supports their decision to make a change. When these inevitable circumstances come up, they don't display adaptability. Instead, they bail. To return to the Lance analogy, they don't learn how to ride in the rain; they just get off the bike and go home. Or more to the point, they pick up a fork and start eating pasta at noon—long before it's time for their workout, which they skip in order to meet their buddies for brewskis after work. When it comes to the Metabolism Advantage plan, the most important thing you can do is this: Stay on the bike!

You see, habits are more powerful than desire. Habits are more powerful than information. Habits are more powerful than guilt. To succeed, you must first make a concerted, committed, conscious effort to override and change your habits.

This chapter will help you do just that. In the coming pages, you will assess your level of preparation with three questionnaires that get at the heart of three important factors in your success. Each questionnaire helps you to definitively answer one of the following three questions.

1. **Are you ready to change?** The first questionnaire will make you look deep within to figure out whether or not you're ready to take your current habits and put them far behind you. If you fill out this questionnaire and decide that you're not ready, it's time for a serious priority shift. After all, we're talking about your metabolism (and your health) here! So use the recommendations in the coming pages and get over to www. MetabolismAdvantage.com for additional advice on how to make this shift.

2. **Is your environment supportive of this change?** In the second questionnaire, you'll take stock of your home and kitchen environment to see if they are conducive to supporting your goals. It always amazes me when people pay lip service to improving their nutrition and health yet don't actually throw out all the bad foods in their kitchens and replace them with good ones. I mean, that's the equivalent of taking an alcoholic who wants to stop drinking and locking him in a room full of liquor.

3. **Is your social circle supportive of this change?** Without adequate social support, changing habits is a losing battle. That said, it's hard to be objective about what our friends bring into our lives, and it's even harder to recognize the friendships that tear us down. This quiz will help you to do that.

Use these questionnaires to assess your readiness to get the Metabolism Advantage. If you score well, you'll have no problem making the changes stick. If you score poorly, you'll find advice throughout this chapter to help you to work on your habits, your environment, and your social circle while taking steps toward increasing your exercise and improving your nutrition.

When taking each quiz, be honest. You're doing these self-assessments to pinpoint areas of your life that might hinder your progress. Resist the urge to guess or to choose the answer that applies to your ideal life. Rather, choose the answer that actually applies to your life as it is today.

Assessment #1: Are You Ready?

In this questionnaire, you'll find out if you're really ready to make the changes needed to boost your metabolism and improve your body composition, health, and physical performance. Answer the questions by circling the one answer most appropriate to your situation. Once you've completed the questions, add up the numbers with the answers you've circled and compare your score to the score key.

1. Do you look in the mirror and get frustrated, upset, or humiliated because of how your body looks?	**A)** Yes (+3) **B)** I'm not sure (0) **C)** No (-3)
2. When you feel rundown and tired, do you blame "getting older," or do you blame your lifestyle habits?	**A)** I blame getting older (-1) **B)** I blame my lifestyle choices (+3) **C)** I blame something else altogether (-3)
3. Are you taking any medications for heart disease, high blood pressure, type 2 diabetes, or another age-related disease that you didn't have when you were younger?	**A)** Yes, I'm on a number of these medications (+3) **B)** Yes, I'm on one of these medications (+1) **C)** No, I'm not on any of these medications (-3)
4. How do you explain the fact that you're in worse shape now than when you were younger?	**A)** I think it's my genetics (-1) **B)** I'm less active (+3) **C)** I think it's a natural consequence of aging (-1) **D)** I don't know why it's happening (0)

5. If you don't have anyone to exercise with regularly, are you willing to look for a physical activity partner?	**A)** Yes (+5) **B)** No (-5)
6. Are you willing to join a gym today?	**A)** Yes (+3) **B)** No (-3)
7. If someone told you that you need to throw away all the foods in your cupboard and go shopping for different foods, foods more appropriate to your goal, would you do it?	**A)** Yes (+5) **B)** No (-5)
8. If *The Metabolism Advantage* presents some information on diet and exercise that contradicts what you currently believe, what approach will you take?	**A)** Keep an open mind and give it a try (+3) **B)** Ask a friend (0) **C)** Ignore the advice and use only the things I agree with (-3)
9. Are you willing to have a meeting with your friends and loved ones to talk about your goals?	**A)** Yes, right away (+5) **B)** Yes, but not just yet (-3) **C)** No (-5)
10. If your work environment presents significant barriers to your sticking with the Metabolism Advantage eating, exercise, and supplement plans, would you consider speaking to your employer about changing some of these conditions or are you willing to find new employment?	**A)** Yes (+5) **B)** No (-5)
11. Are you ready to spend less time with people who offer little or no social support for your goals while spending more time with those who do offer support?	**A)** Yes (+5) **B)** No (-5)
12. Can you accept responsibility for the way your body is today and understand that while your old habits don't make you a bad person, you still need to change them?	**A)** Yes (+5) **B)** No (-5)
13. If a friend or loved one suggests that you don't have what it takes to get into great shape, what will be your response?	**A)** I can do it (+2) **B)** I know I've got to make some changes, but I'll take it one day at a time (+5) **C)** Maybe I can't do it (-5)

14. Are you willing to wake up a bit earlier in the morning and stay up a bit later at night to accomplish your goals?	**A)** Yes (+5) **B)** No (-5)
15. Are you willing to do at least 5 hours of physical activity each week?	**A)** Yes (+5) **B)** No (-5)

SCORE KEY

21 to 63

Revving up your metabolism and changing the way you look, feel, and perform have become very important to you, and you realize that the way you're doing things right now simply isn't cutting it. You're tired of not getting results, and you're tired of the growing waistline, the sluggish metabolism, and the fatigue. Not only are you tired of it, you're also committed to doing something about it—today. Congratulations! Getting to this point takes a lot of work. Now, with the Metabolism Advantage plan, you have all the tools you need at your fingertips. Just follow the strategies laid out in this book and at www.MetabolismAdvantage.com, and you'll get there. You've got the power and you're in control. Go get 'em.

-20 to +20

If you scored in this range, it's important for you to stop thinking and start doing. Yes, you're frustrated with the way things are, but you're afraid that a commitment to something like the Metabolism Advantage program will cause you more hassle and difficulty than just sitting back, doing nothing, and continuing to look and feel the way you do today. You're not alone. Many people fear that a new nutrition and exercise program will cause them pain—more pain than that of losing control of the only body they'll ever have. Step outside your shell and seek out some people who are eating well, exercising, getting results, and having fun doing it. Millions of people are following a healthy lifestyle and loving every minute of it. Don't make the mistake of thinking that they never had difficulties to overcome. At some point in time, each of them had to discard unproductive habits. Once they shed their old ways, they got into the zone. You can do the same. What are you waiting for?

-61 to -21

Are you simply toying with the idea of getting your diet and exercise habits in line with what you know they should be? If you are, this book probably isn't for you. Instead, you need a book of statistics: heart disease statistics, diabetes statistics, stroke statistics, and cancer statistics. If you don't make a change, you're going to be one of those statistics. Think I'm joking? I'm not! With each passing year that you avoid good activity and nutrition habits, your risk of disease increases. As your sluggish metabolism becomes even slower, you'll progressively gain fat, lose muscle, and look much older than your actual age. These are the consequences of remaining indifferent to the meds you're on, the weight you've gained, and the environment you've surrounded yourself with. Don't stay indifferent any longer. Take an honest look at how you've changed (inside and out) and admit that you could use a tune-up. I'm willing to help with the Metabolism Advantage plan. You can find me through www.MetabolismAdvantage.com, but you have to want the help.

Assessment #2: Is Your Environment Supportive Of This Change?

There's a fundamental law of human nutrition that I teach to my clients, and it goes like this: "If a food is in your possession or in your residence, you will eventually eat it. Whether you plan to or not, whether you want to or not, you'll eventually eat it."

Therefore, according to this important law of human nutrition, if you wish to be healthy and lean, you must remove all foods that aren't part of your healthy eating program and replace them with a variety of better, healthier choices.

How do you know which foods have to go and which can stay? Simply read the questions below and circle the answers most appropriate to your situation. Once you've completed the questions, add up the numbers with the answers you've circled and use the score key to understand your score.

| 1. Do you have the following items in your kitchen?
❑ Good set of pots and pans
❑ Good set of knives
❑ Spatula
❑ Blender
❑ Teakettle
❑ Scale for weighing foods
❑ Plastic containers for carrying meals
❑ Small cooler for taking meals to work
❑ Shaker bottle for drinks and shakes
❑ Food processor | A) I have all of them (-5)
B) I have more than half of them (-2)
C) I have fewer than half of them (+2)
D) I don't have any of them (+5) |

2. Do you have the following items in your pantry? ❏ Whole oats ❏ Quinoa ❏ Natural peanut butter ❏ Mixed nuts ❏ Canned or bagged beans ❏ Extra-virgin olive oil ❏ Vinegar ❏ Green tea ❏ Protein supplements ❏ Fish-oil supplements ❏ Greens supplements	**A)** I have all of them (-5) **B)** I have more than half of them (-2) **C)** I have fewer than half of them (+2) **D)** I don't have any of them (+5)
3. Do you have the following items in your fridge or freezer? ❏ Extra-lean (96%) ground beef ❏ Chicken breasts ❏ Salmon ❏ Omega-3 eggs ❏ Packaged egg whites ❏ At least four varieties of fruit ❏ At least five varieties of veggies ❏ Flaxseed oil	**A)** I have all of them (-5) **B)** I have more than half of them (-2) **C)** I have fewer than half of them (+2) **D)** I don't have any of them (+5)
4. Do you have the following items in your pantry? ❏ Potato or corn chips ❏ Fruit or granola bars ❏ Regular or low-fat cookies ❏ Crackers ❏ Regular peanut butter ❏ Chocolates or other candy ❏ Soda ❏ Instant foods like cake mixes and mashed potatoes ❏ Bread crumbs, croutons, or other dried bread products ❏ At least four types of alcohol	**A)** I have all of them (+5) **B)** I have more than half of them (+2) **D)** I have fewer than half of them (-2) **D)** I don't have any of them (-5)

5. Do you have the following items in your fridge or freezer? ❏ At least four types of sauces ❏ Juicy steaks or sausage ❏ Margarine ❏ Fruit juice ❏ Soda ❏ Baked goods ❏ Frozen dinners ❏ At least two types of breads or bagels ❏ Takeout or restaurant leftovers ❏ Big bowl of mashed potatoes or pasta	**A)** I have all of them (+5) **B)** I have more than half of them (+2) **C)** I have fewer than half of them (-2) **D)** I don't have any of them (-5)
6. Do you have bowls of candy, chips, crackers, or other snacks sitting around at home?	**A)** Yes (+5) **B)** No (-5)
7. When you have parties or dinner guests, do you serve them what you think they'll want or what you think is healthy?	**A)** What I think is healthy (-3) **B)** What I think they want (+3)
8. When food shopping, do you buy big economy-size bags or smaller portions?	**A)** More than half of the time, I buy big economy-size bags (+3) **B)** More than half of the time, I buy smaller portions (-3)
9. How often do you grocery shop?	**A)** Less than three times a month (+5) **B)** About once a week (-1) **C)** More than once a week (-5)
10. Do you keep food in plain view around the house?	**A)** Yes (+3) **B)** No (-3)
11. Do you think healthy eating means "low-fat" eating?	**A)** Yes (+2) **B)** No (-2)
12. If someone were to point to a food in your kitchen, would you know whether it was a high-carbohydrate food, a high-protein food, or a high-fat food?	**A)** Yes (-2) **B)** No (+2)
13. Do you prepare meals from cookbooks that contain healthy recipes?	**A)** Most of the time (-5) **B)** About half of the time (0) **C)** Almost never (+5)

14. Do you prepare meals in advance to take with you to work, on day trips, or on vacations?	A) Yes, always (-5) B) More than half of the time (-2) C) Less than half of the time (+2) D) Almost never (+5)
15. Are you hesitant to throw out "unhealthy" leftovers or gift foods that don't fit into your nutritional plan?	A) Yes, I hate throwing food out (+5) B) No, more than half of the time I throw this stuff out (0) C) No, I always throw this stuff out (-5)

SCORE KEY

32 to 63 points

You've scored high on the kitchen-overhaul questionnaire, but that's not a good thing. Your high score means you're not doing so well. In fact, if your kitchen stays in this condition, you'll have better luck winning the lottery than getting results from the Metabolism Advantage program. Since you're in need of an Extreme Kitchen Makeover, here's what to do.

STEP 1. Grab an extra-large shopping bag.

STEP 2. Without thinking about it, open up that bag and toss in every offensive food item from your fridge, freezer, and cupboards. (In case you're not sure which foods to bag, they include all items from questions 4 and 5 of this quiz).

STEP 3. Walk outside, place the bag in your trashcan, wave goodbye, shed a tear, and step away from the trash.

STEP 4. Get to the supermarket immediately and pick up the foods listed in questions 2 and 3 (along with the Metafoods mentioned in Chapter 3).

0 to 31 points

Your kitchen is not the worst I've seen, but it could certainly use some improvement. Take a look at the inventory above and make sure you've got all the items listed in questions 1 through 3 and none of the items from questions 4 and 5. Begin shopping more frequently, eating fresher items, and being more aware of the foods that you're eating and when. Only then will you be equipped for success on the Metabolism Advantage program.

-31 to -1 points

Nice job; you're doing pretty well in the kitchen department. In fact, with a few minor tweaks, your kitchen will be 100 percent ready to go. Revisit the questions above and figure out exactly what it will take to get closer to a perfect score of -63.

-32 to -63 points

Don't let the low score fool you. This quiz works like golf: The lower your score, the better. A negative score means that you don't need much of a makeover. That's great— congratulations on your great kitchen setup! With your kitchen full of great foods (like those listed in questions 2 and 3) and the right appliances, you'll be the envy of your fellow Metabolism Advantage readers. Keep it up!

Assessment #3: Is Your Social Circle Supportive of This Change?

If you have social support, you have a network of people who support your endeavors, contribute positively to your decision-making processes, and offer advice and inspiration when you need help. Various studies suggest that this type of support can help you transcend even the worst environments and accomplish great things. Unfortunately, lack of social support makes it difficult to accomplish even modest goals. Remember this: Who you become 5 years from now has a lot to do with who you choose to spend your time with today.

The following series of questions will help you assess your level of social support. Simply answer the questions by circling the answer most appropriate to your situation. Once you've completed the questions, add up the numbers with the answers you've circled and then use the score key to understand your score.

1. Do the people you spend each day with (at work or at home) follow healthful lifestyle habits such as watching what they eat, exercising regularly, and taking nutritional supplements?	**A)** Yes, most of them do (+3) **B)** About half do and half don't (0) **C)** No, most of them don't (-3)
2. Does your spouse or partner follow healthy lifestyle habits, such as watching what he/she eats, exercising regularly, and taking nutritional supplements?	**A)** Yes, my spouse/partner does (+5) **B)** No, my spouse/partner doesn't (-5) **C)** I don't have a spouse or partner (0)
3. When you want to perform some physical activity, such as going for a workout or taking a hike, is it easy for you to find a partner to go with?	**A)** Yes, it's easy to find a partner (+2) **B)** No, I don't know anyone (0) **C)** No, those around me dislike activity (-2)

4. At your workplace, do your co-workers regularly bring in treats like cookies, doughnuts, and other snacks?	**A)** Yes, they often do (-4) **B)** Yes, but very infrequently (0) **C)** No, they never do (+4)
5. If you go out to eat more than once a week, do the people you dine with order healthful selections?	**A)** Yes, they always do (+2) **B)** Only about half of the time (0) **C)** No, they never do (-2)
6. Do you belong to any clubs (not including a health club), groups, or teams that meet at least twice a week and do some physical exercise?	**A)** Yes, I've been a member for years (+5) **B)** Yes, I've just started (+2) **C)** No, I don't (0)
7. Do you belong to a health club and attend, on average, at least three times a week?	**A)** Yes, I've been a member for years (+2) **B)** Yes, I've just joined (+1) **C)** No, I don't (0)
8. When discussing the Metabolism Advantage plan with friends, do they seem interested, or do they think you're crazy for starting it?	**A)** They're very interested (+2) **B)** They're not interested (0) **C)** They think I'm crazy (-2)
9. Do the people you live with bring home foods that are considered unhealthy or bad for you?	**A)** Always (-5) **B)** Sometimes (-3) **C)** Never (0)
10. Do the people you live with bring home foods that are considered healthy or good for you?	**A)** Always (+5) **B)** Sometimes (0) **C)** Never (-5)
11. Do the people you live with or work with schedule activities for you that interfere with your preestablished exercise time?	**A)** Always; they don't respect my time (-3) **B)** Sometimes; they don't think about it (-1) **C)** Never; they respect this time (+3)
12. Do those around you bring nutrition, exercise, or supplement information to your attention so that you can stay informed about these topics?	**A)** Always (+5) **B)** Sometimes (+2) **C)** Never (0)

SCORE KEY

20 to 38 Points

Congratulations, you have a great support network around you. Of course, that's not all you'll need to succeed with the Metabolism Advantage plan, but it's a great start. Even though you may have scored relatively high on this questionnaire, you still should do your best to support those around you. Social support works both ways. In order to make sure you keep this great group of people around you, you'll have to offer support to them as well.

5 to 19 Points

It looks like you have some social support, but there are a few areas of your life that will present challenges to your quest. Look around you and be aware of workplace, home, and relationship challenges that may stand in your way. Take a mental inventory of each area and come up with creative ways to improve your social environment.

4 to -14 Points

Your social support is lacking and needs a makeover. While some of your environment isn't conducive to your goals, there are some areas that you can latch on to. Based on your quiz answers, figure out which areas are lacking and take steps to fix them. Join a health club, dine with friends committed to health, spend time doing non-food-related things with your other friends, and avoid the doughnut offerings at work. Although it's easy to blame those around you for not being as supportive as you'd like, following the Metabolism Advantage plan is your choice, not necessarily theirs. Instead of blaming them, simply come up with creative and nonantagonistic ways to enlist their support.

-15 to -31 Points

This score is quite low. You have some real problems in your work and home environments as well as in your relationships. I've encountered some people who have succeeded on the Metabolism Advantage plan by going it alone, but not many. Therefore, without some serious changes, your environment will almost certainly make your old habits stick to you like Superglue. Make the following changes.

1. Tell your friends and family of the importance of this change in your life.

2. Get off the couch, head outside, get in your car, and drive to a health club. Pull out a credit card, sign on the dotted line, and become a member. Join a club or group that meets for regular exercise or find a workout partner who is as motivated as you are.

3. It's easy to blame those around you for not being as supportive as you'd like. Instead, come up with creative and nonantagonistic ways to enlist their support. Of course, if it comes to that point, you may have to pick some new friends. Your social group is one of the most important variables in your success.

Set Some Goals—Today

Okay, now you've inventoried your readiness, your environment, and your social group. You know where to make improvements, so it's time to set some goals.

Goal setting is both a science and an art. While most people think that setting goals means just picking something you don't have right now and going for it, there's more to it than that. Use these tips to unlock the power of goal setting.

Set goals that are specific and measurable. "I will look really good naked" doesn't really give you anything measurable or specific to work on. Will you know "good" when you see it? However, "I will lose 15 pounds of body fat" is specific, since it refers to losing one thing—body fat—and it's measurable, since it specifies a number— 15 pounds.

Set goals that are challenging but realistic. Goals must be big enough to inspire you to action but not so big that you get frustrated with the impossibility of accomplishing them. A goal like "I will lose 80 pounds and be on the cover of *Men's Health* magazine" is a bit too lofty for most people. (Sorry I had to be the one to break it to you!) For someone who weighs 160 pounds and has 25 percent body fat, a challenging but realistic goal is something like "I will be 130 pounds and 12 percent body fat after a full year of training."

Set goals with short-term and long-term components. Make small goals applicable today, bigger goals applicable next week, and even bigger goals applicable next month. Save the biggest goals of all for next year. In this way, you'll create mile markers on your road to metabolism-boosting success.

Frame goals around behaviors, not outcomes. Do you know the difference between a behavior goal and an outcome goal? A behavior goal is based on something you can directly control and do yourself, whereas an outcome goal is based on the end product of a series of behaviors.

Unfortunately, most people set outcome goals such as the following.

I will lose 10 pounds in 10 weeks.
I will make $100,000 next year.

While these goals are specific and measurable as well as challenging and realistic, they are outcomes. Outcomes are *beyond your control.* After all, you can't control your fat cells and their rate of fat metabolism just by hoping they'll shrink, and regrettably, you can't force someone to pay you $100,000 a year.

You *can* control your behaviors, however. How do you pick better goals based on behaviors? Try these on for size.

I will exercise for at least 5 hours per week.
I will eat five or six meals each day.
I will eat vegetables with each meal.
I will eat lean protein with each meal.

And, even though it's beyond the scope of this book, let's talk about that financial thing. Here are some more appropriate goals.

I will go back to school and get an advanced degree in my field.
I will spend most of my time on big, high-return projects.
I will improve one aspect of my job performance each day.
I will duplicate the behaviors of others who are making the amount of money I want to make.

In the end, if you make goals out of behaviors (behaviors you can control yourself), your outcome goals (things like your metabolism, body composition, salary, and so on) will fall right in line—without your having to worry about them.

Tell someone about your goals. Once you set specific goals that you're committed to sticking to, tell someone about them right away and ask that person to hold you accountable. If you keep your goals a secret, it will be easier to blow them off. If you have someone holding you accountable to a higher standard, you'll be more likely to get it done.

Okay, now that you have the goal-setting basics, let's set some behavior goals. Follow these steps.

STEP 1. Look over the results of your social support questionnaire, your kitchen inventory, and your readiness questionnaire. Also, think about your current eating and exercise behaviors. Once you have these in your mind, think about the areas that are in need of immediate improvement.

STEP 2. Pick two specific and measurable behavior goals related to these changes. One goal might be eating six meals each day. Another might be eating protein with every meal. These should be things you can accomplish *this week*. Write them down here.

GOAL 1: _____

_____

_____

_____

GOAL 2: _____

_____

_____

_____

STEP 3. Tell someone about your short-term goals. Tell this person what you intend to accomplish and ask this person to hold you accountable for achieving these goals.

Next, let's set some longer-term goals using the same three steps.

STEP 1. Considering the questionnaires you filled out and your current lifestyle habits, think of two specific and measurable behaviors that you can improve upon over the course of *the next few months*. You might aim to discover enough vegetables that you like in order to eat 6 to 10 vegetable servings a day. Or you might decide to buy all the Metabolism Advantage supplements and take them every day.

STEP 2. Write these behavior goals here.

GOAL 3: _____

_____

_____

_____

GOAL 4: _____

_____

_____

_____

STEP 3. Again, tell someone about these goals and ask this person to hold you accountable for them.

Now, let's come up with two desired outcomes that you think will occur as a result of the behavior goals you just established. Keep in mind that these desired outcomes are not your goals! They are things that you hope will happen as a result of accomplishing your behavior goals. Also, choose an outcome that you can measure. Building a faster metabolism is a great goal but not a measurable one unless you have easy access to a biochemistry lab. Yes, of course, this book is all about revving up your metabolism—and you will do just that—but pick something that you can monitor more easily, such as your pants size or waist measurement.

STEP 1. Think of the outcome you'd most like to achieve by the end of 8 weeks on the Metabolism Advantage plan. Write it down here.

DESIRED OUTCOME #1: _____

_____

STEP 2. Think of the outcome you'd most like to achieve by the end of a full year of following the Metabolism Advantage plan.

Write it down here.

DESIRED OUTCOME #2: _____

_____

STEP 3. If you don't achieve your outcomes, reassess where your challenges lie and figure out a new set of behavior goals that will better help you achieve your desired outcomes.

Pursue Your Goals—Now

Once you've set your goals, you are ready to embark on the Metabolism Advantage plan. The first step is taking some time to get your kitchen in Metabolism Advantage shape. It's always a mystery to me how people expect to change their eating habits without changing their cooking and shopping habits. After all, how can you expect to eat better if your fridge and cupboards are full of the wrong foods? Well, Old Mother Hubbard, you can't.

The next chapter will start off by showing you how to do a kitchen overhaul—and then how to turn your list of Metafoods into convenient, delicious meals that will make it easy to stay on the Metabolism Advantage nutrition program.

Then turn to Chapter 8 to find 8 weeks of meal plans and workouts. If you're the type of person who enjoys a no-brainer blueprint to a faster metabolism, in that chapter you'll find just about everything you need to know. On the other hand, if you're the type of person who prefers to customize your program to fit your individual interests, skim over Chapter 8 and then read Chapter 9 in depth. It will tell you how to modify the main Metabolism Advantage program for your personal goals and lifestyle. No matter which method you choose—the no-brainer blueprint or the customized approach—you'll reap fantastic results in 8 short weeks.

$\boxed{7}$

The Metabolism Advantage Recipes

More than 40 convenient, delicious,
metabolism-boosting meals and snacks

In the following pages, you'll find more than 40 delicious, quick-and-easy recipes that will enable you to do two seemingly contradictory things at once: build a great body and eat great-tasting food. That's right. To boost your metabolism, build muscle, and lose fat, you don't need to eat bland food.

Nor do you have to spend hours in your kitchen chopping, straining, juicing, and dehydrating. You don't have to outfit your kitchen with thousands of dollars worth of complex cooking accoutrements (although you will need a few key appliances). You just need the dedication to spend some time in your kitchen every day.

I'll start by giving you a little assistance in getting the right foods into your fridge and cupboards. Use the following lists to get your kitchen in Metabolism Advantage shape. Stock it with these items and watch as your cupboards help your progress instead of hindering it.

Kitchen Support List

The following items will help you quickly prepare and store your Metabolism Advantage cuisine. Pick them up so you won't have to grill your lean meat on your engine block or carry your Super Shakes to work cupped in the palms of your hands.

Countertop grill. You have to grill that protein somewhere. George Foreman and Hamilton Beach make the process easy. Of course, nothing beats a good outdoor gas grill, but for easy, quick kitchen grilling, pick up one of these.

Cooler. You have to store and carry your snacks and midday meal in something. A brown bag just ain't big enough, so pick up a good-size cooler. Coleman makes a few good ones for this purpose.

Blender. Without a blender, you won't be able to make your Super Shakes. Pick up a good one—one that will have no problem with ice cubes or frozen fruit.

Plastic containers. Pick up five small and five large Tupperware-type containers. The small ones are for carrying your meals in your cooler, whether to work or to other functions. Use the large ones to store food in your fridge.

Shaker bottles. Pick up three 1-liter Rubbermaid Chuggable drink containers for your Super Shakes and workout drinks. Don't cheap out on these (although they're only a few bucks). The Rubbermaid bottles have the best seal and will help keep protein stains out of your favorite shirts.

Fridge and Cupboard List

Now it's time to stock your fridge and cupboard. The following lists include all the ingredients you'll need to prepare all of the Metabolism Advantage recipes.

METABOLISM ADVANTAGE METAFOODS

❑ Extra-lean (96%) ground beef
❑ Salmon (fillets and 14¾-ounce can)
❑ Omega-3 eggs (Pilgrim's Pride Eggs Plus or Eggland's Best)
❑ Low-fat, lactose-free plain yogurt
❑ Spinach
❑ Tomatoes
❑ Cruciferous vegetables (broccoli, cabbage, cauliflower)
❑ Avocados

❑ Mixed berries (blueberries, strawberries, cherries, raspberries)
❑ Oranges
❑ Mixed beans (kidney beans, black beans, chickpeas)
❑ Quinoa
❑ Whole oats, large-flake
❑ Mixed nuts (walnuts, almonds, pecans, cashews)
❑ Olive oil
❑ Flaxseed and flaxseed oil
❑ Green tea

SUPPLEMENTS

❑ Fish-oil capsules
❑ Protein supplements (chocolate- and vanilla-flavored Biotest Metabolic Drive super protein shake)

❑ Greens supplements (Greens+)
❑ Creatine
❑ Postworkout recovery drinks (Biotest Surge)

Visit www.MetabolismAdvantage.com to learn where you can find these supplements at the best prices.

Additional Foods

PROTEINS

- Smoked turkey ham or bacon
- Turkey sausage
- 97–98% lean ground turkey breast
- Chicken breast
- Tuna
- Sea bass
- Sea scallops
- Pasteurized egg whites (such as Egg Beaters)

FRUITS AND VEGETABLES

- Mushrooms
- Black olives
- Greek olives
- Onions
- Scallions
- Snow peas
- Red and green bell peppers
- Celery
- Garlic
- Apples
- Carrots
- Cucumbers
- Pineapple
- Bananas
- Kiwifruit
- Raisins
- Lemons
- Green beans
- Jalapeño peppers
- Lime juice
- Iceberg lettuce
- Water chestnuts, canned
- Bean sprouts
- Acorn squash
- Asparagus
- Shallots
- Cabbage
- Artichoke hearts, canned or frozen
- Spicy hot V8 vegetable juice
- Shredded coconut

DAIRY

- Cottage cheese
- Fat-free cream cheese
- Feta cheese
- Mozzarella cheese
- American cheese
- Colby cheese
- Cheddar cheese

GRAINS AND CARBS

- Oat bran
- Wheat berries
- Wheat bran
- Yams

SAUCES AND OILS

- ❏ Olive oil cooking spray
- ❏ Peanut oil
- ❏ Coconut oil
- ❏ Butter or Smart Balance spread
- ❏ Natural peanut butter
- ❏ Peanut sauce
- ❏ Soy sauce
- ❏ Teriyaki sauce
- ❏ Salsa
- ❏ White cooking wine
- ❏ White wine vinegar
- ❏ Apple cider vinegar

SEASONINGS, SPICES, AND HERBS

- ❏ Paprika
- ❏ Cinnamon
- ❏ Cilantro, fresh
- ❏ Mint leaves, fresh
- ❏ Salt
- ❏ Black pepper
- ❏ Oregano, fresh and dried
- ❏ Parsley, fresh
- ❏ Splenda
- ❏ Tahini
- ❏ Ginger, fresh
- ❏ Coriander
- ❏ Basil, fresh and dried
- ❏ Thyme, fresh and dried
- ❏ Cumin
- ❏ Rosemary, fresh
- ❏ Garlic powder
- ❏ Cardamom pods
- ❏ Cayenne pepper
- ❏ Black mustard seeds
- ❏ Saffron
- ❏ Turmeric
- ❏ Chicken bouillon
- ❏ Cocoa powder, unsweetened
- ❏ Chili powder

Cook Up a Faster Metabolism

The Metabolism Advantage recipes use great foods and also try to point you toward the most convenient options. For example, packaged prewashed spinach, canned beans, and other convenient items reduce your prep time, allowing you to make some of these meals in as little as 5 minutes.

In addition to their ease of preparation, these recipes will help you sneak in the Metabolism Advantage Metafoods. Not sure how to fit in three or more weekly servings of quinoa, cruciferous vegetables, avocado, flaxseed, and other Metafoods? Check out the recipes for the shakes, salads, and desserts. Although dishes such as Chocolate

Peanut Butter Bar and Meta Meat Loaf may sound decadent, they contain plenty of fiber and wholesome nutrition. In fact, if you look closely, you'll see that every recipe—no matter how mouthwatering—contains healthful ingredients.

What if you're the type of guy who uses his oven for storage space? Can you succeed on this plan? Of course you can. Throughout this chapter, I've included important pointers that will take you from cooking novice to cooking pro. Don't know how to flip an omelet or separate an egg white from the yolk? You'll find out in the following pages.

Before you start cooking, I do need to mention one caveat. With each recipe, you'll find information on the number of people it serves along with nutritional stats per serving. The optimal serving size, of course, will vary from person to person. A 190-pound man will eat much more than a 120-pound woman, so scale your portions up or down depending on your size and gender. This is particularly important if you're embarking on this plan with your partner. As a general rule, men and women who live together should *not* eat the same portion sizes.

With that said, you're ready to get cooking. When you pair these recipes with the seven Metabolism Advantage nutritional rules you learned in Chapter 4, you can't fail. Visit www.MetabolismAdvantage. com for hundreds more healthy, great-tasting selections.

Metabolism Advantage Breakfasts

The Metabolism Advantage meal plan in Chapter 8 assumes that you'll work out in the evening, which means breakfast must consist of lean protein. In other words, you'll eat a lot of egg whites (with some yolks thrown in for good measure), usually in the form of omelets.

To speed up your prep time, purchase pasteurized egg whites (such as Egg Beaters brand). If you choose to use whole eggs, you must separate the whites from the yolks. To do this, crack the egg, keeping its contents in one half of the shell. Then pour some of the white into a bowl or pan, using the other half of the shell to catch the yolk. Go back and forth between halves until you have all the whites in the bowl or pan. Alternatively, you can crack all the eggs at once into a bowl and fish out the yolks with a spoon.

For omelets, you'll need a good nonstick skillet. If your omelet keeps sticking no matter how you alter your technique or cooking oil application, you probably need a new skillet! To flip the omelet, hold the skillet handle in one hand. Slip a spatula under the omelet with your dominant hand and slide it around the bottom of the omelet, circling the entire perimeter to make sure it isn't sticking. Then lift the skillet, simultaneously flipping the omelet with the spatula. Catch the omelet gently and ease the pan down to the burner.

GREEK OMELET

The spinach in this recipe helps you sneak in two Metafood servings—spinach and omega-3 eggs—during your first meal of the day. The spinach, feta, and olives are a delicious, salty, savory combination. Most diners serve some version of this omelet (sometimes without the olives), so you can still get your Advantage—even if you're on the road.

4 egg whites plus 1 omega-3 egg, beaten
1 handful fresh spinach
$1/2$ handful crumbled feta cheese
$1/4$ cup chopped black olives

Coat a skillet with olive oil cooking spray. Over medium heat, cook the eggs until firm on the underside. Flip the omelet and place the spinach, feta, and olives on top. Once the underside is firm, fold and slide onto a plate.

Makes 1 omelet

PREP TIME: 10 MINUTES

PER OMELET: 332 calories, 32 g protein, 13 g carbohydrates, 8 g fiber, 5 g sugar, 17 g fat (8 g saturated, 7 g monounsaturated, 2 g polyunsaturated, 0.4 g omega-3, 1.1 g omega-6)

SPINACH AND CHEESE OMELET

Fresh spinach works best for this recipe. Buy a bag of prewashed baby spinach to speed up your meal prep.

4 egg whites plus 1 omega-3 egg, beaten
1 handful fresh spinach
1 slice mozzarella cheese

Coat a skillet with olive oil cooking spray. Over medium heat, cook the eggs until firm on the underside. Flip the omelet and place the spinach and cheese on top. Once the underside is firm, fold and slide onto a plate.

Makes 1 omelet

PREP TIME: 10 MINUTES

PER OMELET: 230 calories, 27 g protein, 5 g carbohydrates, 2 g fiber, 2 g sugar, 11 g fat (5 g saturated, 4.5 g monounsaturated, 1 g polyunsaturated, 0.21 g omega-3, 0.77 g omega-6)

ASIAN SCRAMBLED EGGS

This quick-and-easy recipe will liven up your breakfast repertoire. Peanut oil gives this dish a uniquely nutty flavor.

$^1/_2$ cup chopped mushrooms
$^1/_4$ cup chopped onions
5 snow peas, quartered
3 medium scallions, chopped
$^1/_4$ red or green bell pepper, cored, seeded, and chopped
2 teaspoons peanut oil
2 cloves garlic, chopped
1 tablespoon soy sauce
4 egg whites plus 1 omega-3 egg, beaten

In a large skillet over medium heat, cook the mushrooms, onions, snow peas, scallions, bell pepper, oil, garlic, and soy sauce, until soft but still firm. Add the eggs and cook, stirring, for 2 minutes or just until the eggs are cooked.

Makes 1 serving

PREP TIME: 15 MINUTES

PER SERVING: 217 calories, 20 g protein, 13.5 g carbohydrates, 3 g fiber, 4.5 g sugar, 9.5 g fat (2.35 g saturated, 4.1 g monounsaturated, 3.15 g polyunsaturated, 0.25 g omega-3, 2.7 g omega-6)

SCRAMBLED EGGS AND GREENS

This is a staple meal on my breakfast table. There's something about the taste, texture, and nutritive properties of this omelet that really hits the spot first thing in the morning. Fresh spinach works best for this recipe. Buy a bag of prewashed fresh spinach, or be prepared to spend a lot of time over the sink, washing each leaf. If you don't want to bother with fresh spinach, you can use frozen; just thaw and drain it before cooking.

4 ounces smoked turkey ham, chopped
1 handful fresh spinach or $^1/_3$ cup thawed and drained
   frozen spinach
$^1/_2$ cup mushrooms, sliced
$^1/_3$ onion, chopped
6 large egg whites (1 cup) plus 1 omega-3 egg, beaten
1 slice fat-free American cheese

Coat a nonstick skillet with olive oil cooking spray. Over medium-high heat, cook the ham, spinach, mushrooms, and onions for 3 minutes or until the spinach is dark green and condensed. Add the eggs and cheese and cook, stirring, for 2 minutes or just until the eggs are cooked.

Makes 1 serving

PREP TIME: 5 MINUTES

PER SERVING: 408 calories, 58 g protein, 14 g carbohydrates, 4 g fiber, 7 g sugar, 12 g fat (3.6 g saturated, 4.5 g monounsaturated, 2 g polyunsaturated, 0.6 g omega-3, 3 g omega-6)

MEXICAN FRITTATA

This revved-up version of a Central American breakfast includes plenty of tomato, one of your Metafoods. If you're not afraid of a little spice in the morning, add a little hot-pepper sauce for nice zing and an extra metabolism boost.

> 2 ounces lean turkey sausage, sliced, or turkey bacon, crumbled
> $\frac{1}{2}$ small onion, chopped
> $\frac{1}{4}$ red bell pepper, cored, seeded, and chopped
> 3 egg whites plus 1 omega-3 egg, beaten
> 1 medium tomato, chopped
> $\frac{1}{4}$ cup shredded Cheddar cheese
> $\frac{1}{4}$ cup salsa
> 1 teaspoon paprika

Coat a large skillet with olive oil cooking spray. Over medium heat, cook the sausage, onion, and bell pepper for 10 minutes or until the sausage is cooked through. Add the eggs and cook, occasionally lifting the edges to allow the top portion to flow under the lower portion, for 5 to 8 minutes. When the eggs are nearly cooked through, add the tomato, cheese, salsa, and paprika and cook for 5 minutes.

Makes 1 serving

PREP TIME: 20 MINUTES

PER SERVING: 345 calories, 38 g protein, 11 g carbohydrates, 2 g fiber, 6 g sugar, 16 g fat (7 g saturated, 5 g monounsaturated, 3 g polyunsaturated, 0.4 g omega-3, 2.8 g omega-6)

DENVER OMELET

Here's a guilt-free version of a traditional breakfast often served at greasy-spoon diners. This recipe provides a heaping helping of high-quality protein to fuel muscle growth.

> 2 teaspoons butter, coconut oil, or Smart Balance spread
> 4 ounces turkey ham, chopped
> $\frac{1}{2}$ small onion, chopped
> $\frac{1}{2}$ green bell pepper, cored, seeded, and cut into strips
> 6 large egg whites (1 cup) plus 1 omega-3 egg, beaten
> 1 slice fat-free American cheese

Heat 1 teaspoon butter in a large skillet over medium heat. Add the ham and onion and cook until browned. Add the bell pepper and cook for 2 minutes, then transfer to a plate. Add the remaining butter and the eggs to the skillet and cook until firm on the underside. Flip the omelet, then top with the cheese, ham, and vegetables. Fold the omelet over to serve.

Makes 1 omelet

PREP TIME: 20 MINUTES

PER OMELET: 477 calories, 71 g protein, 11 g carbohydrates, 1 g fiber, 7 g sugar, 14 g fat (5 g saturated, 4 g monounsaturated, 5 g polyunsaturated, 0.5 g omega-3, 3.5 g omega-6)

THE BIG OMELET

This omelet will keep you satisfied all morning long.

> 2 teaspoons butter, coconut oil, or Smart Balance spread
> 3 ounces lean turkey sausage, sliced
> 1/4 small onion, chopped
> 1/2 Roma tomato, chopped
> 1/8 cup fresh cilantro, chopped
> 3 egg whites (1/2 cup) plus 1 omega-3 egg, beaten
> 1/4 cup shredded Colby cheese

Heat 1 teaspoon butter in a large skillet over medium heat. Add the sausage and onion and cook until brown. Add the tomato and cilantro and cook, stirring, for 3 minutes or until the tomato becomes soft but is not completely dissolved. Transfer to a plate. Add the remaining butter and the eggs to the skillet and cook until firm on the underside. Flip the omelet, then top with the sausage mixture and cheese. Fold the omelet over to serve.

Makes 1 omelet

PREP TIME: 20 MINUTES

PER OMELET: 480 calories, 53 g protein, 7 g carbohydrates, 1 g fiber, 3 g sugar, 25 g fat (11 g saturated, 8 g monounsaturated, 5 g polyunsaturated, 0.7 g omega-3, 4.3 g omega-6)

Metabolism Advantage Super Shakes

These shakes are all quick-and-easy meals in a glass. All you need is a blender and the ingredients. Each shake features numerous Metabolism Advantage Metafoods, including nuts, flaxseed, yogurt, mixed berries, green tea, and oatmeal. For recipes that call for ground flaxseed, you can either buy whole seeds and grind them in a coffee grinder or simply purchase flax meal.

On the meal plan in Chapter 8, you'll drink a Super Shake every day. If you love one shake in particular, feel free to stick with it. Or, if you prefer more variety, mix and match the shakes as you see fit.

BERRY BLAST

I bet you've never thought about putting oatmeal in a shake before! This Metafood provides blood sugar–stabilizing fiber and helps turn this shake into a thick, satisfying meal.

> 1–1½ cups iced green tea
> 1 scoop vanilla-flavored milk protein blend
> 1 serving Greens+
> 3 tablespoons low-fat, lactose-free plain yogurt
> 3 tablespoons whole oats
> ½ cup frozen mixed berries (including blueberries, strawberries, cherries, and raspberries)

In a blender, combine the tea, protein blend, Greens+, yogurt, and oats and process on high for 1 minute. Add the berries and process for 1 minute.

Makes 1 shake

PREP TIME: 2 MINUTES

PER SHAKE: 259 calories, 30 g protein, 28 g carbohydrates, 6 g fiber, 12.2 g sugar, 3 g fat (1.2 g saturated, 0.2 g monounsaturated, 1.4 g polyunsaturated, 0.1 g omega-3, 0.3 g omega-6)

APPLE AND GREAT GRAINS

This great recipe has healthy grains, fruits, veggies, protein, fiber, and more! It tastes like hearty applesauce.

1–1¹/₂ cups water
1 scoop vanilla-flavored milk protein blend
1 serving Greens+
4 tablespoons ground flaxseed
4 tablespoons whole oats
3 tablespoons low-fat, lactose-free plain yogurt
3 tablespoons mixed nuts
1 apple, cored and sliced
Ground cinnamon to taste

In a blender, combine the water, protein blend, Greens+, flaxseed, oats, and yogurt and process on high for 1 minute. Add the nuts, apple, and cinnamon and process for 1 minute. For an ice-cold shake, add 5 ice cubes and process for 1 minute.

Makes 1 shake

PREP TIME: 2 MINUTES

PER SHAKE: 516 calories, 42 g protein, 62 g carbohydrates, 21 g fiber, 22 g sugar, 29 g fat (4.2 g saturated, 10.8 g monounsaturated, 12.7 g polyunsaturated, 7.1 g omega-3, 4.6 g omega-6)

TWO GREAT TASTES

After drinking this shake, you can check off not one, not two, not three, but four Metafood servings. The chocolate and peanut butter combination makes this shake decadently delicious.

> 1–1½ cups water
> 1 scoop chocolate-flavored milk protein blend
> 1 serving Greens+
> 3 tablespoons low-fat, lactose-free plain yogurt
> 3 tablespoons ground flaxseed
> 3 tablespoons mixed nuts
> 1 tablespoon natural peanut butter

In a blender, combine the water, protein blend, Greens+, yogurt, and flaxseed and process on high for 1 minute. Add the nuts and peanut butter and process for 1 minute. For an ice-cold shake, add 5 ice cubes and process for 1 minute.

Makes 1 shake

PREP TIME: 2 MINUTES

PER SHAKE: 415 calories, 42 g protein, 26 g carbohydrates, 12 g fiber, 6.7 g sugar, 33 g fat (4.9 g saturated, 14 g monounsaturated, 12.8 g polyunsaturated, 5.3 g omega-3, 6.5 g omega-6)

Metabolism Advantage Salads and Veggies

When making salads and veggies, you can either chop by hand or use a food processor. If you chop by hand, use a cleaver, chef's knife, or some other broad-bladed knife. Hold it in your dominant hand and use your other hand to hold down the food, with your fingers pointing straight down. Angle the blade 5 to 10 degrees away from your fingers so that the upper part of the knife rests on your knuckles and the blade touches the cutting surface. Start chopping by sliding the broad side of the knife forward and back without lifting the knife from the cutting board. The flat side of the knife should ride along your knuckles, which should remain upright but slightly bent. Use short, controlled movements. Once you get the hang of it, increase your speed.

METABOLISM ADVANTAGE SALAD

This staple of the Metabolism Advantage meal plan includes plenty of veggies to neutralize dietary acids. It also features six metabolism-boosting Metafoods.

> 1–2 cups spinach
> 1 tomato, sliced
> 1 cup broccoli, chopped
> 1/2 avocado, sliced
> 1/2 cup baby carrots, chopped
> 3 tablespoons mixed nuts
> 3 tablespoons rinsed and drained mixed beans

In a medium bowl, toss together the spinach, tomato, broccoli, avocado, carrots, nuts, and beans. Top with one of the salad dressings on page 182.

Makes 2 servings

PREP TIME: 5 MINUTES

PER SERVING: 245 calories, 11 g protein, 25 g carbohydrates, 15 g fiber, 7 g sugar, 14 g fat (2.3 g saturated, 4.1 g monounsaturated, 1.8 g polyunsaturated, 0.3 g omega-3, 1.6 g omega-6)

SPINACH SAUTÉ

Serve this quick and easy dish with any lunch or dinner to balance out any protein with some tasty vegetables.

> 2 cups spinach
> 1 tomato, sliced
> 1/4 onion, chopped
> 1 clove garlic, chopped

Coat a skillet with olive oil cooking spray. Add the spinach, tomato, onion, and garlic. Cook over low heat, stirring frequently, until the tomato starts to liquefy and the spinach starts to wilt.

Makes 1 serving

PREP TIME: 10 MINUTES

PER SERVING: 135 calories, 14 g protein, 24 g carbohydrates, 15 g fiber, 6.3 g sugar, 2 g fat (0.3 g saturated, 0.1 g monounsaturated, 0.8 g polyunsaturated, 0.5 g omega-3, 0.3 g omega-6)

MEDITERRANEAN SALAD

When you combine cucumbers with tomatoes and olive oil, you get this simple, elegant salad commonly eaten in the often dry, parched areas of the eastern Mediterranean region. Its quick and easy preparation will allow you to work it into the busiest of schedules.

> 1 large cucumber
> 1 large tomato
> 1 tablespoon olive oil
> Dash of salt

Cut the cucumber and tomato into 1/4" cubes. In a medium bowl, toss with the oil and salt. Refrigerate and serve chilled.

Makes 1 serving

PREP TIME: 5 MINUTES

PER SERVING: 98 calories, 2 g protein, 8 g carbohydrates, 2 g fiber, 5 g sugar, 7 g fat (1 g saturated, 5 g monounsaturated, 1 g polyunsaturated, 0.1g omega-3, 0.7 g omega-6)

TOASTED QUINOA SALAD

Native to the Andes highlands, quinoa is a small, globular grain with a great flavor and incredible nutritive properties that probably are a result of its high-altitude home at above 10,000 feet. Fresh cilantro, mint, and lime juice add zest to this dish. Serve it chilled or use it as a bed for grilled fish or chicken.

> $\frac{1}{2}$ cup quinoa
> 1 cup water
> $\frac{1}{2}$ tablespoon chopped fresh ginger
> $\frac{1}{2}$ small jalapeño pepper, seeded, deveined, and chopped (wear gloves when handling)
> $\frac{1}{8}$ teaspoon salt
> $\frac{1}{2}$ cup fresh cilantro, chopped
> $\frac{1}{4}$ cup chopped red onion
> $\frac{1}{8}$ cup fresh mint leaves, chopped
> $\frac{1}{8}$ cup walnuts
> 2 tablespoons lime juice
> 1 teaspoon olive oil

In a skillet over medium heat, cook the quinoa, stirring, for about 6 minutes or until browned. Set aside. In a saucepan over high heat, bring 1 cup water, the ginger, jalapeño, and salt to a rolling boil. Add the quinoa, reduce heat to low, and cook, covered, for 12 minutes or until all or most of the liquid is absorbed. Drain in a fine mesh strainer, then transfer to a medium bowl and fluff with a fork. When cool, add the cilantro, onion, mint, walnuts, lime juice, and oil. Stir until well blended, then refrigerate. Serve chilled.

Makes 2 servings

PREP TIME: 30 MINUTES

PER SERVING: 201 calories, 7 g protein; 32 g carbohydrates, 3 g fiber, 1 g sugar, 11 g fat (0.5 g saturated, 2.5 g monounsaturated, 2 g polyunsaturated, 0.3 g omega-3, 0.8 g omega-6)

GRILLED PEPPERS AND TOMATOES

This quick and easy veggie side dish will complement a host of entrées. Using your creativity, you can change the taste entirely with a different mixture of spices. If you're in an Italian mood, go heavy with the basil and oregano. If Middle Eastern is on the menu, use a little curry and a bay leaf. Either serve this dish warm immediately after cooking, or store it in the fridge and serve it chilled as a salad.

> 1 red or green bell pepper, cored, seeded, and sliced
> 1 tomato, sliced
> $\frac{1}{2}$ onion, sliced
> $\frac{1}{2}$ tablespoon olive oil
> Dash of salt
> Dash of ground black pepper
> Chopped fresh oregano to taste
> Chopped fresh parsley to taste

Coat a nonstick skillet with olive oil cooking spray. Over medium heat, cook the bell pepper, tomato, and onion for 5 to 7 minutes. Transfer to a plate, add the oil, salt, black pepper, oregano, and parsley, and toss to combine.

Makes 1 serving

PREP TIME: 10 MINUTES

PER SERVING: 141 calories, 3 g protein, 19 g carbohydrates, 5 g fiber, 10 g sugar, 7 g fat (1 g saturated, 5 g monounsaturated, 1 g polyunsaturated, 0.1 g omega-3, 0.8 g omega-6)

CARROT SALAD

This is one of my favorite ways to prepare carrots. The salad has a refreshing, light taste, and the pineapple provides a nice textural component that complements the sweetness of the carrots. Carrot salad is particularly well suited as a side dish with beef or as a counterbalance to spicy-hot dishes. You can also serve it as a dessert.

$1/4$ cup raisins
1 cup water
2 or 3 large carrots, grated
$1/4$ cup chopped pineapple
$1/4$ cup low-fat, lactose-free plain yogurt
Dash of salt
Dash of Splenda

In a small bowl, microwave the raisins in 1 cup water on high for 1 minute, then drain. In a medium bowl, combine the raisins, carrots, pineapple, yogurt, salt, and Splenda. Refrigerate and serve chilled.

Makes 2 servings

PREP TIME: 20 MINUTES

PER SERVING: 134 calories, 3 g protein, 30 g carbohydrates, 4 g fiber, 24 g sugar, 1 g fat (0.7 g saturated, 0.3 g monounsaturated, 0.2 g polyunsaturated, 0.1 g omega-3, 0.1 g omega-6)

FRUIT SALAD

In this fruit salad, lemon juice ensures that the bananas won't turn brown when stored in the refrigerator.

$1/3$ pint strawberries, sliced
1 medium banana, sliced
1 large kiwifruit, sliced
1 tablespoon lemon juice
Splenda to taste (optional)

In a large bowl, combine the strawberries, banana, kiwi, lemon juice, and Splenda and toss lightly to mix. Refrigerate and serve chilled.

Makes 1 serving

PREP TIME: 5 MINUTES

PER SERVING: 183 calories, 3 g protein, 45 g carbohydrates, 8 g fiber, 34 g sugar, 1 g fat (0.2 g saturated, 0.1 g monounsaturated, 0.3 g polyunsaturated, 0.1 g omega-3, 0.2 g omega-6)

HUMMUS

This Levantine dish is a mixture of mashed chickpeas (also called garbanzo beans), garlic, lemon, and tahini. Despite these basic ingredients, the taste and texture of hummus varies widey across regions and even from restaurant to restaurant. Typically, the farther you get from its homeland, the worse hummus tastes. (The canned stuff here in the West shouldn't even be called by the same name.) The precise proportions of ingredients in this recipe produce a hummus worthy of the dinner table in any eastern Mediterranean home.

6 cloves garlic, minced
1 tablespoon + 1/3 cup olive oil
5 tablespoons tahini
Juice of 2 large lemons
1/3 teaspoon salt
3 cans (19 ounces each) chickpeas, rinsed and drained

In a medium skillet over medium heat, cook the garlic in 1 tablespoon oil for 3 to 5 minutes or until browned. In a large food processor, combine the garlic, remaining oil, tahini, lemon juice, salt, and 1 cup chickpeas and process until mashed. Continue adding chickpeas 1 cup at a time until all are processed, adding a small amount of water when the mixture becomes too dry. Process until smooth and creamy. Transfer to a plate or shallow bowl and flatten into a circular shape with a well in the middle. Drizzle olive oil into the well and use the hummus as a dip for your favorite vegetables.

Makes 10 servings

PREP TIME: 20 MINUTES

PER SERVING: 266 calories, 7 g protein, 30 g carbohydrates, 6 g fiber, 4 g sugar, 13 g fat (2 g saturated, 8 g monounsaturated, 3 g polyunsaturated, 0.1 g omega-3, 0.7 g omega-6)

MIXED-BEAN SALAD

This delicious dish is a great way to get in one of your bean servings. You can use either drained and rinsed canned beans or cooked dried beans.

$1/2$ cup green beans
$1/4$ cup mixed beans
1 tomato, chopped
$1/4$ onion, chopped
1 tablespoon olive oil
Salt and ground black pepper to taste
Chopped fresh oregano to taste
Chopped fresh parsley to taste

In a medium bowl, combine the green beans, mixed beans, tomato, onion, oil, salt, pepper, oregano, and parsley. Toss lightly and refrigerate. Serve chilled.

Makes 1 serving

PREP TIME: 5 MINUTES

PER SERVING: 254 calories, 6.4 g protein, 25 g carbohydrates, 10 g fiber, 7 g sugar, 14.7 g fat (2.0 g saturated, 10.8 g monounsaturated, 1.4 g polyunsaturated, 0.2 g omega-3, 1.3 g omega-6)

GUACAMOLE

As long as you skip the corn chips, guacamole is a very healthy source of monoun-saturated fat. This version combines avocados, tomatoes, and lemon juice for a healthy side dish or spread. Instead of dipping chips, try carrots, celery, cucumbers, or any vegetable of your choice. You can also spread guacamole over a roasted chicken breast or fish.

3 medium avocados, peeled and cored
1 medium tomato, chopped
1 teaspoon fresh lemon juice
$1/4$ teaspoon salt

In a large bowl, combine the avocados, tomatoes, lemon juice, and salt. Combine thoroughly, leaving some chunks of avocado for good texture.

Makes 5 servings

PREP TIME: 5 MINUTES

PER SERVING: 190 calories, 2 g protein, 9 g carbohydrates, 5 g fiber, 2 g sugar, 18 g fat (3 g saturated, 12 g monounsaturated, 2 g polyunsaturated, 0 g omega-3, 2.0 g omega-6)

METABOLISM ADVANTAGE TABBOULEH

This low-carb version of the traditional healthful, nutritious Mediterranean salad is an excellent accompaniment to most meals and a great way to incorporate some leafy greens and monounsaturated fats into your diet.

8 **scallions, chopped**
2 **tomatoes, chopped**
1 **cucumber, chopped**
2 **cups fresh parsley, chopped**
$\frac{1}{2}$ **cup fresh mint leaves, chopped**
$\frac{1}{2}$ **cup fresh lemon juice**
1 **clove garlic, chopped**
4 **tablespoons olive oil**
   Salt and ground black pepper to taste

In a large bowl, combine the scallions, tomatoes, cucumber, parsley, mint, lemon juice, garlic, oil, salt, and pepper. Toss until combined.

Makes 6 servings

PREP TIME: 5 MINUTES

PER SERVING: 125 calories, 2 g protein, 10 g carbohydrates, 3 g fiber, 5 g sugar, 10 g fat (1 g saturated, 7 g monounsaturated, 1 g polyunsaturated, 0.1 g omega-3, 0.9 g omega-6)

MASHED GARLIC CAULIFLOWER

This low-carb version of "mashed potatoes" helps you sneak in a serving of cruciferous vegetables to round out your Metafood list.

1 **large head cauliflower**
1 **tablespoon butter, coconut oil, or Smart Balance spread**
2 **cloves garlic, chopped**
1 **teaspoon salt**

In a large saucepan with a tight-fitting lid, steam the cauliflower in 2 inches of boiling water for 15 minutes. Transfer to a food processor in small batches and puree. Add the butter, garlic, and salt and puree until smooth and creamy.

Makes 3 servings

PREP TIME: 25 MINUTES

PER SERVING: 100 calories, 6 g protein, 15 g carbohydrates, 7 g fiber, 6 g sugar, 4 g fat (1 g saturated, 1 g monounsaturated, 2 g polyunsaturated, 0.4 g omega-3, 0.8 g omega-6)

Metabolism Advantage Dressings

The following two Metabolism Advantage dressings can accompany the Metabolism Advantage Salad (page 175). Feel free to alternate between the two or just use the one you like best. The first dressing features olive oil as a source of healthful monounsaturated fats. The second includes flaxseed oil for metabolism-boosting omega-3 fatty acids.

I LOVE OLIVE

Here's a healthy salad dressing that tastes great and is good for you. Ditch the Thousand Island in favor of Popeye's girl.

1 tablespoon extra-virgin olive oil
1 tablespoon white wine vinegar
Chopped fresh basil to taste
Chopped fresh oregano to taste
Salt and ground black pepper to taste

In a small bowl, combine the oil, vinegar, basil, oregano, salt, and pepper and mix with a fork.

Makes 2 servings

PREP TIME: 2 MINUTES

PER SERVING: 126 calories, 0 g protein, 0 g carbohydrates, 0 g fiber, 0 g sugar, 14 g fat (1.9 g saturated, 10.8 g monounsaturated, 1.3 g polyunsaturated, 0.1 g omega-3, 1.1 g omega-6)

FLAX YOUR DRESSING

This healthy dressing also tempts your taste buds and uses flaxseed oil instead of olive oil.

1 tablespoon plain or flavored (garlic and chili) flaxseed oil
1 tablespoon apple cider vinegar
1 teaspoon ground flaxseed
Salt and ground black pepper to taste

In a small bowl, combine the oil, vinegar, flaxseed, salt, and pepper and mix with a fork.

Makes 2 servings

PREP TIME: 2 MINUTES

PER SERVING: 136 calories, .65 g protein, 1.4 g carbohydrates, 0.9 g fiber, 0 g sugar, 14.6 g fat (1.4 g saturated, 2.6 g monounsaturated, 10.1 g polyunsaturated, 8.1 g omega-3, 1.9 g omega-6)

Metabolism Advantage Lunches and Dinners

The numerous salmon and lean beef recipes on the following pages will help you meet your quota for these Metafoods without feeling as if you are eating the same thing over and over again. Because the meal plan in Chapter 8 suggests you use your leftovers from dinner for the next day's lunch, most recipes serve two. Scale them up or down depending on your family size and needs.

You'll also find plenty of chicken dishes. Chicken breast is lean, relatively cheap, and very versatile. It goes well with almost every grain, vegetable, spice, and fruit. On your day off, roast several breasts and then add them to dishes during the week (or eat them for lunch) to reduce your prep time for workday evening meals. Store them in a self-sealing plastic bag or a plastic container in the fridge for up to 3 days. Although 4-day-old chicken is probably safe to eat, it can start to become rubbery.

To roast boneless, skinless chicken breasts, preheat the oven to 400°F. Place the breasts about 1 inch apart on a baking sheet covered with foil. Sprinkle with lemon juice, salt, garlic powder, and black pepper (or use your favorite spice blend) and roast for 30 minutes. Let cool for 15 to 30 minutes before storing them in the fridge. Cook bone-in breasts at 375°F for 45 minutes.

Chapter 8's meal plan also suggests roasted salmon as an occasional alternative to chicken. To roast salmon, preheat the oven to 275°F. Place one or more 5-ounce fillets skin side down on a baking sheet covered with foil. Rub the top of the fish with olive oil, salt, and fresh ground pepper. Cook for 15 to 35 minutes or until the fish separates easily from the skin and a fork inserted straight down into the flesh meets no resistance. When slow roasting, it is common for the top of the cooked fish to appear raw or slightly translucent.

TERIYAKI LETTUCE WRAP

This healthy version of a spring roll is a convenient stand-alone, low-carb meal. Although iceberg lettuce offers little in the way of nutrition, its crisper texture works well for the wrap.

3 **cloves garlic, minced**
2 **tablespoons white cooking wine**
2 **tablespoons teriyaki sauce or soy sauce**
1 **pound boneless, skinless chicken breast, minced**
1 **tablespoon peanut oil**
1 **cup water chestnuts, slivered**
9 **large leaves iceberg lettuce**
1 **cup bean sprouts**

In a medium bowl, combine the garlic, wine, and teriyaki sauce. Add the chicken and let stand for 5 to 10 minutes. Heat the oil in a skillet over medium-high heat. Add the chicken and marinade and cook, stirring constantly, for 5 minutes. Add the water chestnuts and cook for 5 minutes or until the chicken is no longer pink.

Transfer the chicken mixture to a large plate and serve the lettuce and bean sprouts separately. Make the wraps as you eat them by placing the chicken mixture and sprouts in the middle of a lettuce leaf and then rolling the lettuce into a spring roll shape.

Makes 3 servings

PREP TIME: 25 MINUTES

PER SERVING: 250 calories, 37 g protein, 8 g carbohydrates, 2 g fiber, 1 g sugar, 7 g fat (1 g saturated, 3 g monounsaturated, 2 g polyunsaturated, 0.1 g omega-3, 1.8 g omega-6)

CITRUS CHICKEN–STUFFED ACORN SQUASH

Acorn squash has a unique sweet, nutty, peppery flavor. In addition to containing cancer-fighting phytonutrients, it is packed with vitamins such as beta-carotene, vitamin C, vitamin B_1 (thiamin), vitamin B_3, vitamin B_6, folate, pantothenic acid, and potassium. This version of stuffed squash is delicious, very healthy, and even nice to look at.

  2 **medium acorn squash**
  1 **pound boneless, skinless chicken breast, cut into 1-inch cubes**
  2 **medium onions, chopped**
  2 **large stalks celery, sliced into $^1/_4$-inch pieces (1 cup)**
$^1/_2$ **teaspoon salt**
$^1/_2$ **teaspoon ground black pepper**
$^1/_2$ **teaspoon dried thyme**
  1 **tablespoon freshly grated orange peel**

Preheat the oven to 375°F. Cut the squash in half, scoop out the seeds and membranes, and discard. Place squash halves cut side down in a baking dish and add water until it covers $^1/_4$ inch of the squash. Bake for 45 minutes or until fork-tender. (For quick cooking, microwave on high, covered and without the water, for about 10 minutes or until fork-tender.)

Meanwhile, in a nonstick skillet, combine the chicken, onions, celery, salt, pepper, and thyme. Cook over medium-high heat, stirring occasionally, for 15 to 20 minutes or until the chicken is no longer pink. Stir in the orange peel and cook, stirring occasionally, for 3 to 4 minutes or until heated through. To serve, fill each squash half with $^1/_4$ of the chicken mixture.

Makes 2 servings

PREP TIME: 1 HOUR FOR OVEN COOKING; 20 MINUTES FOR MICROWAVE COOKING

PER SERVING: 597 calories, 76 g protein, 56 g carbohydrates, 9 g fiber, 17 g sugar, 9 g fat (3 g saturated, 3 g monounsaturated, 3 g polyunsaturated, 0.1 g omega-3, 1.6 g omega-6)

ROASTED CHICKEN WITH ROSEMARY WHEAT BERRIES

Whole wheat grains, commonly known as wheat berries, have a nutty, wholesome flavor. They also have more vitamins, fiber, and micronutrients than their more processed cousins. Most bulk food bins at whole foods markets have wheat berries at very reasonable prices.

You can cook this dish in bulk, refrigerate it, and then reheat it for a quick meal.

- 4 **cups water**
- 1 **cup wheat berries**
- 2 **cups broccoli florets**
- 2 **cups baby carrots, sliced**
- 2 **tablespoons chopped fresh rosemary**
- 1/2 **teaspoon garlic powder**
  Salt and ground black pepper to taste
- 1 **pound roasted chicken breast, cut into strips**

In a saucepan with a tight-fitting lid, bring 4 cups water and a dash of salt to a boil over high heat. Add the wheat berries, reduce heat to low, and cook, covered, for 45 minutes. Stir in the broccoli, carrots, rosemary, garlic powder, salt, and pepper and cook, covered, for 15 minutes. Uncover and boil off any remaining liquid. Divide the wheat berries and vegetables between 2 plates and top with the chicken.

Makes 2 servings

PREP TIME: 1 HOUR

PER SERVING: 743 calories, 88 g protein, 76 g carbohydrates, 13 g fiber, 6 g sugar, 10 g fat (3 g saturated, 3 g monounsaturated, 3 g polyunsaturated, 0.2 g omega-3, 2.2 g omega-6)

QUICK QUINOA AND CHICKEN

This recipe combines quinoa, chicken breast, spinach, and lemon juice for a flavorful, convenient meal. Spinach and quinoa make a great combination, which is only natural considering that quinoa grows on a leafy, spinach-like plant.

- 1/2 **cup quinoa**
- 8 **ounces roasted chicken breast, cut into 1-inch cubes**
  Large handful fresh spinach
- 2 **tablespoons fresh lemon juice**
  Dash of salt

Cook the quinoa according to the package directions. Coat a large skillet with olive oil cooking spray. Add the chicken and spinach and cook over medium heat for 5 to 7 minutes or just until warm and the spinach reduces and becomes pliable. Transfer the quinoa to a plate and top with the chicken and spinach. Add the lemon juice and salt just before serving.

Makes 1 serving

PREP TIME: 5 MINUTES

PER SERVING: 733 calories, 86 g protein, 67 g carbohydrates, 9 g fiber, 2 g sugar, 14 g fat (3 g saturated, 4 g monounsaturated, 4 g polyunsaturated, 0.3 g omega-3, 1.5 g omega-6)

FAJITA CHICKEN AND RICE

Fajitas have a healthy base (chicken and vegetables), but they are often cooked in unhealthy oils. This recipe skips the tortillas and uses grilled chicken and vegetables as a topping for a bed of spiced brown rice.

  1 **cup brown rice**
 $^1/_2$ **cup salsa**
  1 **teaspoon paprika**
 $^1/_8$ **teaspoon ground cumin**
  1 **pound roasted chicken breast, cut into strips**
  1 **small onion, sliced**
  1 **red or green bell pepper, cored, seeded, and sliced**
     Salt and ground black pepper to taste
  2 **tablespoons lime juice**

Cook the rice according to package directions. In a large bowl, combine the rice, salsa, paprika, and cumin and stir until mixed. Reheat in the microwave for 1 to 2 minutes or on the stove over medium heat for 5 minutes. Coat a large skillet or wok with olive oil cooking spray and add the chicken, onion, and bell pepper. Cook over high heat for 5 minutes or until the onion starts to brown, then add the salt and black pepper. Divide the rice between 2 plates, top with the chicken and vegetables, and drizzle with the lime juice.

Makes 2 servings

PREP TIME: 10 MINUTES

PER SERVING: 750 calories, 79 g protein, 80 g carbohydrates, 5 g fiber, 5 g sugar, 11 g fat (3 g saturated, 4 g monounsaturated, 3 g polyunsaturated, 0.2 g omega-3, 2.5 g omega-6)

CHICKEN WITH CHICKPEAS

Chickpeas, which are included among the mixed beans on the list of Metafoods, are full of nutrients and fiber. When combined with chicken, they create the perfect blend of nutrients for your day off from the gym or sometime outside the workout window, when you want to limit carbs.

> 2 teaspoons olive oil
> 2 cloves garlic, chopped
> 8 ounces roasted chicken breast, chopped
> $\frac{1}{2}$ onion, chopped
> 1 can (15$\frac{1}{2}$ ounces) chickpeas, rinsed and drained
> 1 large tomato, chopped
> $\frac{1}{4}$ teaspoon ground cumin
> $\frac{1}{4}$ teaspoon salt
> 2 cardamom pods

Heat 1 teaspoon oil in a large skillet over medium heat. Add the garlic and cook, stirring frequently, for 2 to 4 minutes. Add the chicken and onion and cook, stirring constantly, for 3 to 5 minutes or until the onion begins to brown. Add the chickpeas, tomato, cumin, salt, and cardamom and cook, stirring, for 5 minutes longer, until the mixture begins to thicken.

Makes 2 servings

PREP TIME: 10 MINUTES

PER SERVING: 485 calories, 49 g protein, 45 g carbohydrates, 13 g fiber, 5 g sugar, 12.5 g fat (2 g saturated, 5 g monounsaturated, 3 g polyunsaturated, 0.1 g omega-3, 1.2 g omega-6)

COCONUT CHICKEN WITH BROCCOLI

Saturated fat, often considered a "bad" fat associated with heart disease, does have a place in your diet—as long as it's balanced with monounsaturated and polyunsaturated fats. This recipe uses coconut, a plant source of saturated fat and one generally recognized as having many health-promoting properties. The coconut forms a flaky crust for the chicken and is complemented by steamed broccoli with olive oil and lemon juice.

Chicken

- ²/₃ cup shredded coconut
- 3 cloves garlic, chopped
- 2 tablespoons butter, coconut oil, or Smart Balance spread
- 1¹/₂ pounds boneless, skinless chicken breasts (about 2 large breasts)

Broccoli

- 3 cups chopped broccoli
- 2 tablespoons fresh lemon juice
- 2 teaspoons olive oil
- Salt and ground black pepper to taste

To make the chicken: Preheat the oven to 400°F. Coat a baking sheet with olive oil cooking spray. In a medium bowl, combine the coconut, garlic, and butter. Microwave on low until the butter softens, then stir well and spread evenly onto the top of the chicken. Place on the baking sheet and bake for 10 minutes, then set the oven to broil and broil for 10 minutes.

To make the broccoli: Meanwhile, put 1 inch of water in a large saucepan and bring to a boil over high heat. Add the broccoli and cook for 8 to 10 minutes. Transfer to a plate and top with the lemon juice, olive oil, salt, and pepper.

Makes 2 servings

PREP TIME: 30 MINUTES

PER SERVING: 713 calories, 86 g protein, 26 g carbohydrates, 8 g fiber, 14 g sugar, 29 g fat (14 g saturated, 7 g monounsaturated, 5 g polyunsaturated, 0.5 g omega-3, 3.5 g omega-6)

BAKED YAM AND TURKEY MEATBALL MARINARA

Yams are a great source of fiber and nutrient-rich carbohydrates, making this meal perfect after a workout. Thankfully, you can quickly nuke them and stuff them with pre-made ingredients.

3 medium tomatoes, chopped

8 cloves garlic, chopped

2 medium onions, chopped

1 large green bell pepper, cored, seeded, and sliced

Dash of dried oregano

Dash of dried basil

Salt to taste

1 pound 97–98% lean ground turkey breast

1 omega 3 egg, beaten

Ground black pepper to taste

1 medium yam

Preheat the oven to 400°F. In a nonstick skillet over medium-low heat, combine the tomatoes, half of the garlic, half of the onions, the bell pepper, oregano, basil, and a dash of salt. Stir and cover.

In a large bowl, combine the turkey, the remaining garlic and onion, the egg, a dash of salt, and the black pepper. Form into 2-inch meatballs, place on a baking sheet, and bake for 15 to 20 minutes or until the juices run clear.

With a fork or knife, poke some holes in the yam. Microwave on high for 6 minutes or until you can easily insert a fork into the center.

In a large bowl, combine the meatballs and tomato sauce. Cut the yam down the center and mash the flesh with a fork. Stuff with the meatballs and sauce and microwave until warm.

Makes 2 servings

PREP TIME: 30 MINUTES

PER SERVING: 553 calories, 64 g protein, 64 g carbohydrates, 11 g fiber, 14 g sugar, 4 g fat (1 g saturated, 1 g monounsaturated, 2 g polyunsaturated, 0.2 g omega-3, 1.1 g omega-6)

SALMON BURGER STROGANOFF

Canned salmon is convenient, but it takes some creativity and preparation to make it palatable. Most salmon burger recipes produce a dry, tasteless meal, but the mushroom sauce makes this one a mouthwatering delicacy.

Burgers

1 large can (14³/₄ ounces) salmon
1 tablespoon fresh lemon juice
1 omega-3 egg, beaten
¹/₂ small onion, diced
¹/₄ cup flax meal
¹/₄ cup oat bran
¹/₈ teaspoon turmeric
Salt and ground black pepper to taste

Sauce

1 tablespoon butter or Smart Balance spread
2 cups sliced mushrooms
3 cloves garlic, minced
1 chicken bouillon cube
¹/₄ cup water
5 tablespoons whole plain yogurt

To make the burgers: Drain the salmon, reserving 1 tablespoon of liquid. Place the salmon and liquid in a large bowl, then remove the larger bones from the salmon and discard. Add the lemon juice and mix. Add the egg, onion, flax meal, oat bran, turmeric, salt, and pepper and mix thoroughly. Shape and flatten into 2 large patties. Coat a skillet with olive oil cooking spray. Add the patties and cook over medium heat for 8 to 10 minutes on each side.

To make the sauce: Heat the butter in a skillet over medium heat. Add the mushrooms and garlic and cook, stirring frequently, for 6 to 8 minutes or until browned. Add the bouillon and 1/4 cup water and bring to a gentle boil. Stir in the yogurt 1 tablespoon at a time until smooth and creamy. Top the burgers with sauce just before serving.

Makes 2 servings

PREP TIME: 30 MINUTES

PER SERVING: 514 calories, 53 g protein, 21 g carbohydrates, 6.4 g fiber, 4.8 g sugar, 26 g fat (6.7 g saturated, 6.3 g monounsaturated, 8.3 g polyunsaturated, 5.9 g omega-3, 1.9 g omega-6)

ROSEMARY SALMON AND ASPARAGUS ON THE GRILL

Given its meaty composition, salmon is great on the grill. This recipe combines the powerful fragrance and flavor of rosemary with the great properties of salmon. Asparagus completes this dish that is surprisingly easy to make.

2 tablespoons fresh lemon juice
1 tablespoon olive oil
3 cloves garlic, chopped
2 tablespoons fresh rosemary, chopped
Salt and ground black pepper to taste
1 pound salmon fillets, cut into 2 pieces
20 large asparagus spears, trimmed

Preheat the grill to medium-high. In a small bowl, combine the lemon juice, oil, garlic, rosemary, salt, and pepper. Place the salmon skin side down on a piece of foil large enough to wrap completely around the fillets. Brush with the lemon juice mixture and fold the foil around the salmon, leaving a small (1 inch) hole at the top. Grill with the lid closed for 10 to 15 minutes or until either the center is slightly pink (if the salmon is very fresh) or the fish is white and flaky throughout (if you're not sure about the freshness).

About 5 minutes after beginning to cook the fish, coat the asparagus with olive oil, then place on the grill lengthwise so the spears don't slip through the grate. Every other minute or so, roll the spears to prevent charring. When the asparagus is browned (after 5 to 10 minutes), salt lightly and remove from the grill. When the fish is done, remove the skin, which will stick to the foil.

Makes 2 servings

PREP TIME: 20 MINUTES

PER SERVING: 533 calories, 50 g protein, 12 g carbohydrates, 5 g fiber, 4 g sugar, 32 g fat (6 g saturated, 14 g monounsaturated, 10 g polyunsaturated, 4.6 g omega-3, 4.6 g omega-6)

SALMON IN BASIL CREAM SAUCE

This recipe uses yogurt rather than heavy cream to meld with the other ingredients, creating full-flavored harmony that will satisfy your taste buds.

1	pound salmon fillets, cut into 2 pieces and skin removed
2 or 3	shallots, chopped
2	cloves garlic, minced
$1/3$	cup white cooking wine
$3/4$	cup fresh basil, chopped
$1/8$	cup fresh parsley, chopped
$1/8$	teaspoon salt
	Juice of 1 large lemon
$1/2$	cup whole plain yogurt

In a skillet over medium-high heat, sear the salmon for 3 minutes on each side. Transfer to a plate. (The centers of the fillets may not be completely cooked, which is fine because the fish will continue to cook after you remove it from the skillet.)

In the same skillet over medium-low heat, cook the shallots and garlic for 5 minutes or until golden brown. Increase the heat to medium-high and add the wine, basil, parsley, salt, and lemon juice. Bring to a boil, then slowly stir in the yogurt 1 to 2 tablespoons at a time and cook until the sauce is reduced by half. Add the salmon and reheat. To serve, spoon the sauce over the salmon.

Makes 2 servings

PREP TIME: 30 MINUTES

PER SERVING: 628 calories, 54 g protein, 12 g carbohydrates, 1 g fiber, 5 g sugar, 37 g fat (8 g saturated, 16 g monounsaturated, 11 g polyunsaturated, 5.2 g omega-3, 4.9 g omega-6)

PECAN-CRUSTED SALMON

Pecan meal and olive oil create an aromatic crust for salmon, complementing the omega-3 fatty acids in the fish with a healthy dose of monounsaturated fat. To make the pecan meal, process the nuts in a blender on low, 1 cup at a time. Refrigerate in an airtight container. Steamed spinach rounds out this meal.

> 2 **tablespoons pecan meal**
> 1 **teaspoon olive oil**
> 10 **ounces salmon fillet**
> **Salt and ground black pepper to taste**
> 2 **big handfuls (about 20 mature leaves) spinach**

Preheat the oven to 400°F. Line a baking sheet with foil.

In a small bowl, mix the pecan meal and oil, then press the salmon into the mixture to coat the top. Sprinkle with the salt and pepper and place skin side down on the baking sheet. Bake for 6 minutes, then set the oven to broil and broil for 6 minutes. Remove from the oven and separate the fish from the skin, which will stick to the foil.

Meanwhile, place 1 inch of water in a large saucepan and bring to a boil over high heat. Add the spinach and cook for 5 minutes.

Makes 1 serving

PREP TIME: 15 MINUTES

PER SERVING: 680 calories, 57 g protein, 9 g carbohydrates, 7 g fiber, 1 g sugar, 47 g fat
(8 g saturated, 20 g monounsaturated, 15 g polyunsaturated, 5.7 g omega-3, 8.6 g omega-6)

GREEK BURGER, FOREMAN STYLE

Thanks to a George Foreman–style countertop grill, this meal will take just 5 minutes to prepare and cook. That's about how long you'd have to stand in line at your favorite fast-food joint to get a much less healthful burger.

> 1 **pound extra-lean (96%) ground beef**
> ½ **cup crumbled feta cheese**
> ½ **cup black olives, sliced**
> 3 **cloves garlic, chopped**
> **Salt and ground black pepper to taste**

In a large bowl, combine the beef, cheese, olives, garlic, salt, and pepper. Form into 2 large patties and grill for 5 minutes.

Makes 2 servings

PREP TIME: 5 MINUTES

PER SERVING: 600 calories, 77 g protein, 5 g carbohydrates, 1 g fiber, 2 g sugar, 29 g fat
(12 g saturated, 12 g monounsaturated, 1 g polyunsaturated, 0.1 g omega-3, 1.0 g omega-6)

TUNA BURGERS

You can turn plain old canned tuna into a delicious meal by adding just a few ingredients. Flax meal and omega-3 eggs form a nice matrix for these burgers and add metabolism-boosting omega-3 fatty acids. Serve this dish with Grilled Peppers and Tomatoes (page 177) or Toasted Quinoa Salad (page 176).

> 3 **cans (14 ounces each) water-packed chunk light tuna, drained**
> 4 **scallions, minced**
> 2 **omega-3 eggs, beaten**
> 2 **cloves garlic, chopped**
> 1/4 **cup flax meal**
> 2 **tablespoons black mustard seed**
> 1 **tablespoon finely minced fresh cilantro**
> 1 **teaspoon soy sauce**
>   **Salt and ground black pepper to taste**
> 2 **teaspoons olive oil**

In a large bowl, combine the tuna, scallions, eggs, garlic, flax meal, mustard seed, cilantro, soy sauce, salt, and pepper. Form into 2 patties. Heat the oil in a large skillet over medium heat. Add the burgers and cook for about 6 minutes on each side or until browned on both sides and cooked through.

Makes 2 servings

PREP TIME: 20 MINUTES

PER SERVING: 475 calories, 63 g protein, 14 g carbohydrates, 7 g fiber, 2 g sugar, 18 g fat
(3 g saturated, 9 g monounsaturated, 6 g polyunsaturated, 3.2 g omega-3, 2.4 g omega-6)

ALMOND-CRUSTED SEA SCALLOPS WITH TOMATO-ONION GRATIN

Sea scallops provide a large dose of protein with very little fat. For this meal, almonds and olive oil supply healthy monounsaturated fats. This dish is a real crowd pleaser.

Gratin

2 medium tomatoes, cut into ¼-inch-thick wedges
1 medium onion (preferably Vidalia), sliced
⅓ cup grated Parmesan cheese
2 cloves garlic, chopped
2 teaspoons olive oil
Salt and ground black pepper to taste

Scallops

½ cup almonds
1½ pounds sea scallops, rinsed and patted dry
½ teaspoon salt
¼ teaspoon cayenne pepper
1 tablespoon olive oil
¼ cup fresh cilantro, coarsely chopped

To make the gratin: Preheat the oven to 450°F. Coat an 8" x 8" baking dish with olive oil cooking spray. In a large bowl, toss together the tomatoes, onion, cheese, garlic, oil, salt, and pepper. Spread evenly in the baking dish and bake for 25 minutes.

To make the scallops: Meanwhile, in a blender, grind the almonds into a coarse meal. Spread on a dinner plate. Sprinkle the scallops with salt and cayenne, then press them into the almonds, coating all sides and shaking off the excess.

Heat 1½ teaspoons oil in a large skillet over medium-high heat. Add only enough scallops to cover the bottom of the skillet in a single layer and cook for 2 minutes on each side or until browned and crisp. Transfer to a plate and cook the remaining scallops, adding the remaining oil as needed. To serve, arrange on top of the gratin and garnish with the cilantro.

Makes 2 servings

PREP TIME: 30 MINUTES

PER SERVING: 717 calories, 73 g protein, 23 g carbohydrates, 6 g fiber, 7 g sugar, 37 g fat (6 g saturated, 22 g monounsaturated, 7 g polyunsaturated, 0.8 g omega-3, 5.5 g omega-6)

SEARED SCALLOPS IN SPINACH CREAM SAUCE

Use this protein-rich meal to appease any significant other who grumbles about your eating habits. It's simple, delicious, full of micronutrients, and suitable for a candlelit dinner with a fine wine.

    1 **package (6 ounces) sliced mushrooms**
    3 **cloves garlic, diced**
    4 **tablespoons diced shallots or 8 chopped scallions**
       1-inch cube fresh ginger, diced
    1 **pound sea scallops**
    2 **packages (10 ounces each) frozen spinach, thawed**
    8 **tablespoons whole plain yogurt**
    2 **large carrots, sliced**
    2 **tablespoons fresh lemon juice**
       Pinch of saffron or dash of turmeric
       Salt and ground black pepper to taste

Coat a skillet with olive oil cooking spray and heat over medium heat. Add the mushrooms, garlic, shallots, and ginger and cook, stirring frequently, for 2 minutes. Add the scallops and cook for 2 to 3 minutes or until opaque. Add the spinach and bring to a boil. Add the yogurt 1 tablespoon at a time, stirring it in evenly. Add the carrots, lemon juice, saffron, salt, and pepper and cook, stirring frequently, for 15 to 20 minutes. (Some of the liquid should boil off, but if the mixture starts becoming dry, cover the skillet for the remainder of the cooking time.)

Makes 2 servings

PREP TIME: 30 MINUTES

PER SERVING: 413 calories; 56 g protein; 40 g carbohydrates; 14 g fiber; 9 g sugar; 5 g fat (2 g saturated; 1 g monounsaturated; 2 g polyunsaturated; 0.8 g omega-3; 0.4 omega-6)

STRIPED BASS WITH ARTICHOKE AND ASPARAGUS

Slow baking at low heat in the oven creates an incredibly tender and moist bass fillet. White wine, garlic, and black olives complement striped bass without overshadowing it.

Fish

> 1   **teaspoon olive oil**
> 2   **cloves garlic, thinly sliced**
> 1½ **pounds striped bass fillets**
> 4   **tablespoons sliced Greek olives**
> 1½ **tablespoons dry white wine**
>   **Salt and ground black pepper to taste**

Vegetables

> 1   **can (14 ounces) artichoke hearts, drained**
> 1   **tablespoon olive oil**
> 2   **cloves garlic**
> 1   **pound asparagus, trimmed and cut into 2-inch lengths**
> ¼   **cup water**
> ⅓   **cup fresh parsley, chopped**
>   **Salt and ground black pepper to taste**
> 1   **lemon, halved**

To make the fish: Preheat the oven to 225°F. Lightly brush the oil on the bottom of a baking dish just large enough to hold the fish. Scatter the garlic in the dish, then add the fish, skin side down. Top with the olives, drizzle with the wine, and sprinkle with the salt and pepper. Bake for 15 to 20 minutes or until the fish separates easily from the skin and a kitchen fork slides easily into the thickest part.

To make the vegetables: Soak the artichokes in cold water for 15 to 20 minutes to remove the brine taste. While the fish is cooking, combine the oil and garlic in a large skillet over medium-high heat. Add the artichokes, increase the heat to high, and cook, stirring constantly, for 4 minutes or until starting to brown. Add the asparagus and ¼ cup water. Cover and cook for 2 to 4 minutes, tossing occasionally. Uncover and let any remaining water evaporate. Add the parsley, salt, and pepper. Transfer to a plate, squeeze the juice of the lemon over the top, and serve as a bed for the fish.

Makes 2 servings

PREP TIME: 25 MINUTES

PER SERVING: 528 calories, 68 g protein, 22 g carbohydrates, 10 g fiber, 5 g sugar, 20 g fat (3 g saturated, 11 g monounsaturated, 4 g polyunsaturated, 2.7 g omega-3, 1.1 g omega-6)

THAI GROUND BEEF

The cabbage in this recipe allows you to sneak in a serving of cruciferous veggies—one of your Metabolism Advantage Metafoods.

> 4 ounces extra-lean (96%) ground beef
> 3 cups shredded cabbage
> 1/2 carrot, sliced
> 1/2 medium green bell pepper, cored, seeded, and cut into 1-inch cubes
> 1/2 small onion, cut into 1-inch cubes
> 1 tablespoon peanut sauce
> Chili powder to taste
> Salt and ground black pepper to taste

Coat a large nonstick skillet with olive oil cooking spray and heat over medium-high heat. Add the beef and cook, stirring frequently, for 5 minutes or until browned. Add the cabbage, carrot, bell pepper, and onion and cook, stirring frequently, for 5 minutes or until browned. Add the peanut sauce, chili powder, salt, and black pepper.

Makes 2 servings

PREP TIME: 20 MINUTES.

PER SERVING: 574 calories, 77 g protein, 18 g carbohydrates, 6 g fiber, 9 g sugar, 21 g fat (6 g saturated, 9 g monounsaturated, 3 g polyunsaturated, 0.2 g omega-3, 2.9 g omega-6)

CHILI IN A FLASH

Thanks to canned beans and V8, this recipe is the fastest chili dish around. The cashews add a unique element that helps you meet one of your Metafood requirements. Look for them at a health food store.

 1 **pound extra-lean (96%) ground beef**
 ¹/₂ **onion, chopped**
 1 **yellow bell pepper, cored, seeded, and cut into ¹/₂-inch squares**
 1 **can (15¹/₂ ounces) kidney beans, rinsed and drained**
 1 **cup spicy hot V8 vegetable juice cocktail**
 ¹/₂ **cup cashews**
 1 **packet chili seasoning**

In a large nonstick skillet or wok, cook the ground beef and onion on high heat for 3 minutes or until browned. Add the bell pepper and cook, stirring, for 1 minute. Stir in the beans, vegetable juice cocktail, cashews, and seasoning and bring to a boil. Reduce the heat to low and cook for 15 to 30 minutes.

Makes 2 servings

PREP TIME: 5 MINUTES

PER SERVING: 637 calories, 71 g protein, 53 g carbohydrates, 11 g fiber, 18 g sugar, 13 g fat (4 g saturated, 6 g monounsaturated, 2 g polyunsaturated, 0.1 g omega-3, 1.1 g omega-6)

EXTRA-LEAN BEEF MEATBALLS

You'll sneak flaxseed into this classic dish to meet one of your Metafood requirements. The wheat bran not only helps hold the meatballs together but also adds a dose of fiber to the dish.

 5 **ounces extra-lean (96%) ground beef**
 1 **omega-3 egg + 1 omega-3 egg white, beaten**
 2 **cloves garlic, chopped**
 ¹/₄ **small onion, finely chopped**
 ¹/₈ **cup ground flaxseed**
 ¹/₈ **cup wheat bran**
  Salt and ground black pepper to taste

Preheat the oven to 375°F. Coat a baking sheet with olive oil cooking spray. In a large bowl, combine the beef, egg, garlic, onion, flaxseed, bran, salt, and pepper. Form the mixture into 2" meatballs (about 4 or 5). Place on the baking sheet and bake for 30 minutes or until a toothpick inserted in the center of a meatball comes out clean.

Makes 1 serving

PREP TIME: 45 MINUTES

PER SERVING: 475 calories, 46 g protein, 15 g carbohydrates, 9.5 g fiber, 2 g sugar, 25.5 g fat (7.6 g saturated, 9.2 g monounsaturated, 5.6 g polyunsaturated, 3.6 g omega-3, 1.5 g omega-6)

META MEAT LOAF

This recipe discreetly includes cottage cheese without anyone other than the chef knowing it's there. With slow-digesting carbs and fiber from the oat bran and omega-3s from flaxseed, this is probably the healthiest meat loaf you'll ever eat.

1 **pound extra-lean (96%) ground beef**
2 **stalks celery, chopped**
1 **omega-3 egg, beaten**
1 **medium onion, finely chopped**
1 **clove garlic, crushed**
1 **cup low-fat cottage cheese**
$1/_2$ **cup oat bran**
$1/_4$ **cup chopped seeded green bell pepper**
2 **tablespoons whole flaxseed or 4 tablespoons ground flaxseed**
$1/_2$ **teaspoon salt**
$1/_4$ **teaspoon ground black pepper**

Preheat the oven to 350°F. Coat a 9" x 5" loaf pan with olive oil cooking spray. In a large bowl, combine the beef, celery, egg, onion, garlic, cottage cheese, bran, bell pepper, flaxseed, salt, and pepper. Spread the mixture into the baking dish and bake for 45 minutes.

Makes 2 servings

PREP TIME: 50 MINUTES

PER SERVING: 548 calories, 69 g protein, 32 g carbohydrates, 9 g fiber, 8 g sugar, 19 g fat (6 g saturated, 7 g monounsaturated, 5 g polyunsaturated, 2.4 g omega-3, 2.2 g omega-6)

Metabolism Advantage Snacks

Snacks and bars are certainly optional—no one's going to hold a gun to your head and force you to eat them. That said, you won't need a lot of prodding, because these sweet treats are just as delicious as they are good for your metabolism. They're also quick and easy to prepare.

If you're going to keep treats in your kitchen, make them these and not Twinkies, chocolate chip cookies, and other foods with absolutely no fiber and little in the way of nutrition. Each of the following features one or more of the Metabolism Advantage Metafoods along with a good dose of fiber. Collectively, they are the healthiest desserts you'll ever love.

NO-BAKE STRAWBERRY CHEESECAKE

Although this treat is delicious, the oat bran and flaxseed help to ensure that it's also good for you—and your metabolism.

Crust

- 1 **cup graham cracker crumbs**
- $1/4$ **cup ground flaxseed**
- $1/4$ **cup oat bran**
- 1 **ounce fat-free cream cheese, warmed in microwave**

Filling

- 2 **cups low-fat cottage cheese**
- $1/2$ **package (52 grams) Jell-O instant pudding mix, cheesecake flavor**
- 3 **ounces fat-free cream cheese**
- 3 **scoops vanilla-flavored milk protein blend**
- 2 **cups sliced strawberries**

To make the crust: Coat a 9" pie pan with olive oil cooking spray. In a large bowl, combine the graham cracker crumbs, flaxseed, bran, and cream cheese. Stir until it is an even consistency, then press into the pie pan, stretching the crust up the sides.

To make the filling: In a blender, combine the cottage cheese, pudding mix, cream cheese, and protein blend. Blend on high until smooth and creamy and stir in the strawberries. Pour into the crust and refrigerate for 1 hour.

Makes 4 servings

PREP TIME: 25 MINUTES

PER SERVING: 408 calories, 58 g protein, 14 g carbohydrates, 4 g fiber, 7 g sugar, 12 g fat (3.6 g saturated, 4.5 g monounsaturated, 3.9 g polyunsaturated, 0.59 g omega-3, 3 g omega-6)

CHOCOLATE PEANUT BUTTER BAR

Satisfy your taste buds while you consume Metabolism Advantage Metafoods. To make the pecan and almond meal, process the nuts in a blender on low, 1 cup at a time. Refrigerate in an airtight container.

6 scoops chocolate-flavored milk protein blend
1 omega-3 egg + 1 omega-3 egg white, beaten
$^1/_2$ cup pecan meal
$^1/_2$ cup almond meal
$^1/_2$ cup natural peanut butter
$^1/_3$ cup flax meal
$^1/_4$ cup Splenda
1 tablespoon unsweetened cocoa powder
$^1/_4$ teaspoon salt

Preheat the oven to 350°F. Coat an 8" x 8" baking dish with olive oil cooking spray. In a large bowl, combine the protein blend, egg, pecan meal, almond meal, peanut butter, flax meal, Splenda, cocoa, and salt. If the mixture becomes too coarse, add some water 1 tablespoon at a time until moistened. Spread into the baking dish and bake for 6 to 12 minutes, checking frequently to make sure the bars do not dry out. (If in doubt, err on the side of underdone rather than overdone. Even underdone, they're a tasty treat.)

Makes 6 bars

PREP TIME: 20 MINUTES

PER BAR: 396 calories, 33 g protein, 12 g carbohydrates, 5 g fiber, 4 g sugar, 26 g fat (4 g saturated, 13 g monounsaturated, 8 g polyunsaturated, 1.1 g omega-3, 6.5 g omega-6)

8

The Metabolism Advantage Planner

Your 8-week blueprint to a faster metabolism

Welcome to the Metabolism Advantage planner. In the following pages, you'll find everything you need to follow the Metabolism Advantage plan for 8 weeks. For each of the following 55 days, you'll find Metabolism Advantage workouts and menu suggestions. There's even space to keep track of your results and plan for the upcoming week.

This planner makes three important assumptions.

1. You work a Monday-to-Friday 9-to-5ish job.
2. You prefer to work out in the evening during the week and in the morning on Saturdays.
3. You'd like to take a day off from exercise on Sunday.

Why do these assumptions matter? In Chapter 4, you learned about the importance of nutrient timing. According to this concept, your muscles are most receptive to absorbing carbohydrate during and just after your workouts. That means that if you work out in the evening, you should consume a carbohydrate-rich recovery drink during and after your workout and include carbohydrate in your meal soon afterward. It also means that you *do not* necessarily want to eat high-carbohydrate meals earlier in the day, when your muscle cells are less receptive to absorbing them.

Assuming you work out in the evening on weekdays, you'll have grains, starchy vegetables, or fruit for dinner but not for breakfast or lunch. I assumed that you would prefer to work out in the mornings on Saturdays, so on these days, the planner calls for you to consume grains, fruit, and other carb-rich foods for breakfast.

What if you prefer to work out at a different time of day? Can you still use this planner? Of course you can. Just eat your carbs at a different time. For example, if you work out in the morning, substitute some whole grain toast with your postworkout breakfast in place of eating the quinoa suggested for dinner. If you work out at midday, have some quinoa, rice, or fruit with lunch in place of the grain suggested with dinner. No matter when you exercise, always have a carbohydrate-rich recovery drink during and after your workout.

What if you're the type of person who likes to go it alone? Do you have to use this planner to succeed on the program? Absolutely not. If you want to come up with your own meal plan—based on the rules you learned in Chapter 4—and pair it with the workouts you learned in Chapter 5 (or others you'll find in Chapter 9), go for it!

Otherwise, let me be your guide. Each day of this planner includes between five and seven meals and snacks. Don't let all the food suggestions overwhelm you. In many cases, some of the meals are no more complicated than opening a bottle of your favorite recovery drink and inserting it into your mouth. You'll also find many easy shake and salad suggestions. Most of the breakfast and lunch options (and even some dinner options) take just 5 minutes or less to prepare.

For optimal success, use these pointers.

- Scale the meal portions up or down depending on your gender, body size, and personal genetics. In the pages that follow, you'll find a one-size-fits-all meal plan. Just as with one-size-fits-all clothing, this plan may be too big or too small for you. Each day of the plan provides roughly 2,600 to 3,400 calories. For most men, that's about right. For some men and many women, however, that's probably too much food. In that case, you'll probably want to scale back on many of the suggested meal portions. Let your stomach be your guide. Once you feel satisfied, stop eating. Don't force yourself to eat an entire portion just because it's sitting in front of you!
- Each Sunday, look over the menus for the week to come. Use Sundays as prep days. Shop for the ingredients you'll need for the upcoming week. Cook up extra chicken breasts to use for lunches and dinners that call for them. Chop up the veggies you'll need for various salad dishes. Put your workouts on your calendar.
- Splurge as needed. Remember the 90 percent rule that I mentioned earlier? Well, I've *planned* it into your menus. Each week, you'll find up to four meals and snacks that simply say, "10 percent." Use them as opportunities to eat out or have your favorite foods.
- Make the most of leftovers. A number of the lunches on these menus use fish, chicken, and other foods left over from the night before. Also, many of the recipes serve two, so if you're single, you'll have leftovers. Use those in place of other meals on busy days. If you have a family, however, you'll need to double or triple the recipes, depending on the number of mouths you're feeding, in order to have some left over for the next day.
- Many of the meals and recipes use quick-and-easy convenience foods. In all cases, you can follow recipes in the previous chapter. That said, some specialty stores sell some of these ingredients (such as roasted peppers, grilled veggies, or hummus) already

prepared. Feel free to use them as long as they're prepared in a similar manner to the meals here. The more convenient you make the plan, the more likely you'll be to stick with it.

- Keep records. For your strengthening workouts, the plan provides space for you to write down the weight you used and number of reps you completed. Use this space! Recordkeeping not only keeps you motivated—by helping you to easily see your progress—but also helps you better plan for your next workout. If you completed seven or eight reps of an exercise that calls for just five reps, for example, you'll know you need to increase the weight for your next workout.

- Start the program on a Monday, the very next one!

Week 1

SHOPPING LIST

DRY GOODS

- ❑ 3 cans (15½ ounces each) mixed beans (kidney beans, black beans, chickpeas)
- ❑ 1 can (15½ ounces) sliced black olives, preferably Greek
- ❑ 1 can (8 ounces) juice-packed pineapple chunks
- ❑ 1 can (14 ounces) artichoke hearts
- ❑ 1 box (9 ounces) raisins
- ❑ 1 pound oat bran
- ❑ 1 pound wheat bran
- ❑ Shelled mixed nuts (1 pound each walnuts, almonds, pecans, cashews)
- ❑ 1 pound quinoa
- ❑ 1 bag (1 or 2 pounds) whole flaxseed
- ❑ At least 16 cups' worth green tea

PRODUCE

- ❑ 1½ pounds fresh spinach
- ❑ 4 oranges
- ❑ 1 green apple
- ❑ 1 pint strawberries
- ❑ 1 medium banana
- ❑ 1 large kiwifruit
- ❑ 3 large lemons
- ❑ 2 limes
- ❑ 9 tomatoes
- ❑ 4 medium white onions
- ❑ 1 red onion
- ❑ 3 medium scallions
- ❑ 1 small jalapeño or 1 can (4 ounces) sliced jalapeños
- ❑ 1 large cucumber
- ❑ 2-inch piece fresh ginger
- ❑ 2 green bell peppers
- ❑ 1 bunch celery
- ❑ 1 pound asparagus
- ❑ 1 pound broccoli
- ❑ 3 avocados
- ❑ 4 ounces mushrooms
- ❑ 10 snow peas
- ❑ 1 pound baby carrots
- ❑ 3 large carrots
- ❑ 1 head cabbage
- ❑ 2 or 3 shallots
- ❑ 4 ounces fresh or frozen green beans
- ❑ 1 head garlic
- ❑ 1 bunch fresh cilantro
- ❑ 1 bunch fresh mint
- ❑ 1 bunch fresh parsley
- ❑ 1 bunch fresh basil

REFRIGERATED ITEMS

- ❏ 4 ounces feta cheese
- ❏ 2 containers (32 ounces each) pasteurized egg whites (such as Egg Beaters)
- ❏ 1 dozen omega-3 eggs (Pilgrim's Pride Eggs Plus or Eggland's Best)
- ❏ 8 ounces low-fat cottage cheese
- ❏ 4 ounces fat-free American cheese, sliced
- ❏ 8 ounces shredded Cheddar cheese
- ❏ 1 container (8 ounces) low-fat, lactose-free plain yogurt
- ❏ 8 ounces butter, coconut oil, or Smart Balance spread

MEATS

- ❏ 2½ pounds salmon fillets
- ❏ 1½ pounds striped sea bass, with skin
- ❏ 1½ pounds extra-lean (96%) ground beef
- ❏ 4 ounces turkey ham
- ❏ 2 ounces turkey sausage or turkey bacon
- ❏ 1½ pounds boneless, skinless chicken breasts

CONDIMENTS, OILS, SPICES, MISCELLANEOUS

- ❏ Ingredients for 13 Metabolism Advantage Super Shakes of your choice (page 172)
- ❏ Ingredients for 1 Snack or Bar (page 202)
- ❏ 2 containers (32 ounces each; approximately 10 servings) recovery drink
- ❏ Fish-oil capsules
- ❏ Ingredients for 10 percent meal
- ❏ Olive oil
- ❏ Peanut oil
- ❏ Soy sauce
- ❏ Peanut sauce
- ❏ Chili powder
- ❏ Dried oregano
- ❏ Paprika
- ❏ Salt
- ❏ Ground black pepper
- ❏ Dried basil
- ❏ Tabasco sauce
- ❏ Splenda
- ❏ Worcestershire sauce
- ❏ 1 jar (16 ounces) salsa
- ❏ Cooking wine
- ❏ Dry white wine

Once you've assembled the food you'll need for Week 1, get started. Good luck!

DAY 1: MONDAY

Meal Plan

MEAL 1: Greek Omelet (page 167), 1 orange, 1 or 2 fish-oil capsules, 1 cup green tea

MEAL 2: Any Metabolism Advantage Super Shake (pages 172), 1 or 2 fish-oil capsules, ½ teaspoon creatine

MEAL 3: 5-ounce roasted salmon fillet, Metabolism Advantage Salad (page 175) with either Metabolism Advantage dressing (page 182), 1 or 2 fish-oil capsules

MEAL 4: Any Metabolism Advantage Super Shake (page 172), 1 or 2 fish-oil capsules, ½ teaspoon creatine

MEAL 5 (DURING WORKOUT): ½ recovery drink

MEAL 6 (POSTWORKOUT AT 7 PM): ½ recovery drink

MEAL 7: Meta Meat Loaf (page 201), Spinach Sauté (page 175), 1 or 2 fish-oil capsules, 1 cup green tea

Lower-Body Strengthening Workout (page 99)

5-MINUTE CARDIOVASCULAR WARMUP:	Bicycling, walking, rowing, or stairclimbing
BARBELL SQUAT: 2 sets of 5–7 reps	Set 1: ___ lb ___ reps Set 2: ___ lb ___ reps
OVERHEAD BARBELL SQUAT: 2 sets of 5–7 reps	Set 1: ___ lb ___ reps Set 2: ___ lb ___ reps
BARBELL DEADLIFT: 3 sets of 5–7 reps	Set 1: ___ lb ___ reps Set 2: ___ lb ___ reps Set 3: ___ lb ___ reps
DUMBBELL WALKING LUNGE: 2 sets of 5–7 reps with each leg	Set 1: ___ lb ___ reps per leg Set 2: ___ lb ___ reps per leg
SINGLE-LEG SWISS BALL LEG CURL: 2 sets of 5–7 reps with each leg	Set 1 (right leg): ___ reps Set 1 (left leg): ___ reps Set 2 (right leg): ___ reps Set 2 (left leg): ___ reps
STEPUP: 2 sets of 5–7 reps on each side	Set 1: ___ lb ___ reps per side Set 2: ___ lb ___ reps per side
5-MINUTE CARDIOVASCULAR COOLDOWN:	Bicycling, walking, rowing, or stairclimbing

◼ DAY 2: TUESDAY

WEEK 1

MEAL 1: Denver Omelet (page 170), ½ avocado, 1 or 2 fish-oil capsules, 1 cup green tea

MEAL 2: Any Metabolism Advantage Super Shake (page 172), 1 or 2 fish-oil capsules, ½ teaspoon creatine

MEAL 3: Leftover Meta Meat Loaf from previous day, Mixed-Bean Salad (page 180), 1 or 2 fish-oil capsules

MEAL 4: Any Metabolism Advantage Super Shake (page 172), 1 or 2 fish-oil capsules, ½ teaspoon creatine

MEAL 5 (DURING WORKOUT): ½ recovery drink

MEAL 6 (POSTWORKOUT): ½ recovery drink

MEAL 7: Salmon in Basil Cream Sauce (page 193), Toasted Quinoa Salad (page 176), 1 or 2 fish-oil capsules, 1 cup green tea

Interval Workout #1

5-MINUTE LOW-INTENSITY WARMUP

INTERVALS: Perform 7 total intervals
30 seconds at high intensity,
90 seconds at low intensity

5-MINUTE LOW-INTENSITY COOLDOWN

■ DAY 3: WEDNESDAY

Meal Plan

MEAL 1: Spinach and Cheese Omelet (page 168), 1 orange, 1 or 2 fish-oil capsules, 1 cup green tea

MEAL 2: Any Metabolism Advantage Super Shake (page 172), 1 or 2 fish-oil capsules, ½ teaspoon creatine

MEAL 3: Chunks of leftover Basil Salmon from previous day, sprinkled on Metabolism Advantage Salad (page 175) with either Metabolism Advantage dressing, 1 or 2 fish-oil capsules

MEAL 4: Any Metabolism Advantage Super Shake (page 172), 1 or 2 fish-oil capsules, ½ teaspoon creatine

MEAL 5 (DURING WORKOUT): ½ recovery drink

MEAL 6 (POSTWORKOUT): ½ recovery drink

MEAL 7: 10 percent meal, 1 or 2 fish-oil capsules, 1 cup green tea

Upper-Body Strengthening Workout (page 105)

5-MINUTE CARDIOVASCULAR WARMUP:	Bicycling, walking, rowing, or stairclimbing
BENT-OVER BARBELL ROW: 3 sets of 5–7 reps (2 sets with overhand grip, 1 set with underhand grip)	Set 1 (overhand grip): ___ lb ___ reps Set 2 (overhand grip): ___ lb ___ reps Set 3 (underhand grip): ___ lb ___ reps
FLAT BARBELL BENCH PRESS: 3 sets of 5–7 reps (1 set with medium grip, 1 set with wide grip, 1 set with narrow grip)	Set 1 (medium grip): ___ lb ___ reps Set 2 (wide grip): ___ lb ___ reps Set 3 (narrow grip): ___ lb ___ reps
PULLUP: 2 sets of 5–7 reps	Set 1: ___ reps Set 2: ___ reps
BARBELL OVERHEAD PRESS: 2 sets of 5–7 reps	Set 1: ___ lb ___ reps Set 2: ___ lb ___ reps
SINGLE-ARM BARBELL BICEPS CURL: 2 sets of 5–7 reps with each arm	Set 1 (right arm): ___ reps Set 1 (left arm): ___ reps Set 2 (right arm): ___ reps Set 2 (left arm): ___ reps
DIP: 2 sets of 5–7 reps	Set 1: ___ reps Set 2: ___ reps
5-MINUTE CARDIOVASCULAR COOLDOWN:	Bicycling, walking, rowing, or stairclimbing

■ DAY 4: THURSDAY

Meal Plan

MEAL 1: Asian Scrambled Eggs (page 168), 1 green apple, 1 or 2 fish-oil capsules, 1 cup green tea

MEAL 2: Any Metabolism Advantage Super Shake (page 172), 1 or 2 fish-oil capsules, ½ teaspoon creatine

MEAL 3: Roasted chicken breast, Mediterranean Salad (page 176), 1 or 2 fish-oil capsules

MEAL 4: Any Metabolism Advantage Super Shake (page 172), 1 or 2 fish-oil capsules, ½ teaspoon creatine

MEAL 5 (DURING WORKOUT): ½ recovery drink

MEAL 6 (POSTWORKOUT): ½ recovery drink

MEAL 7: Pecan-Crusted Salmon (page 194), Toasted Quinoa Salad (page 176), 1 or 2 fish-oil capsules, 1 cup green tea

Interval Workout #2

5-MINUTE LOW-INTENSITY WARMUP

INTERVALS: Perform 7 total intervals
60 seconds at high intensity,
60 seconds at low intensity

5-MINUTE LOW-INTENSITY COOLDOWN

■ DAY 5: FRIDAY

Meal Plan

MEAL 1: Greek Omelet (page 167), 1 orange, 1 or 2 fish-oil capsules,
1 cup green tea

MEAL 2: Any Metabolism Advantage Super Shake (page 172),
1 or 2 fish-oil capsules, $\frac{1}{2}$ teaspoon creatine

MEAL 3: Leftover Pecan-Crusted Salmon from previous day, crumbled on
Metabolism Advantage Salad (page 175) with either Metabolism
Advantage dressing (page 182), 1 or 2 fish-oil capsules

MEAL 4: Any Metabolism Advantage Super Shake (page 172),
1 or 2 fish-oil capsules, $\frac{1}{2}$ teaspoon creatine

MEAL 5 (DURING WORKOUT): $\frac{1}{2}$ recovery drink

MEAL 6 (POSTWORKOUT): $\frac{1}{2}$ recovery drink

MEAL 7: Quick Quinoa and Chicken (page 186), Carrot Salad (page 178),
Fruit Salad (page 178), 1 cup green tea

Total-Body Strengthening Workout (page 111)

5-MINUTE CARDIOVASCULAR WARMUP:	Bicycling, walking, rowing, or stairclimbing
PUSHUP ON SWISS BALL: 2 sets of 8–10 reps	Set 1: ___ reps Set 2: ___ reps
SUITCASE DEADLIFT: 3 sets of 8–10 reps on each side	Set 1 (right side): ___ lb ___ reps Set 1 (left side): ___ lb ___ reps Set 2 (right side): ___ lb ___ reps Set 2 (left side): ___ lb ___ reps Set 3 (right side): ___ lb ___ reps Set 3 (left side): ___ lb ___ reps
BARBELL CLEAN: 3 sets of 8–10 reps	Set 1: ___ lb ___ reps Set 2: ___ lb ___ reps Set 3: ___ lb ___ reps
DUMBBELL OVERHEAD WALKING LUNGE: 2 sets of 8–10 reps with each leg	Set 1: ___ lb ___ reps per leg Set 2: ___ lb ___ reps per leg
BRIDGE: 2 sets of 30 seconds each	Set 1: ___ Set 2: ___
SIDE BRIDGE: 2 sets of 30 seconds on each side	Set 1 (right side): ___ Set 1 (left side): ___ Set 2 (right side): ___ Set 2 (left side): ___
5-MINUTE CARDIOVASCULAR COOLDOWN:	Bicycling, walking, rowing, or stairclimbing

■ DAY 6: SATURDAY (ASSUMING AM WORKOUT)

Meal Plan

MEAL 1 (DURING WORKOUT): ½ recovery drink

MEAL 2 (POSTWORKOUT): ½ recovery drink

MEAL 3: Mexican Frittata (page 170), ½ avocado or Guacamole (page 180), 1 or 2 fish-oil capsules, 1 cup green tea

MEAL 4: Any Metabolism Advantage Super Shake (page 172), 1 or 2 fish-oil capsules, ½ teaspoon creatine

MEAL 5: Thai Ground Beef (page 199), Toasted Quinoa Salad (page 176), Mixed-Bean Salad (page 180), 1 or 2 fish-oil capsules

MEAL 6: 10 percent meal, 1 or 2 fish-oil capsules, 1 cup green tea

MEAL 7: Any Metabolism Advantage Super Shake (page 172), 1 or 2 fish-oil capsules, ½ teaspoon creatine

Interval Workout #3

5-MINUTE LOW-INTENSITY WARMUP

INTERVALS:	Perform 4 total intervals
90 seconds at high intensity, 180 seconds at low intensity	

5-MINUTE LOW-INTENSITY COOLDOWN

■ DAY 7: SUNDAY (ASSUMING NO WORKOUT)

Meal Plan

MEAL 1: 10 percent meal, 1 or 2 fish-oil capsules, 1 cup green tea

MEAL 2: Extra-Lean Beef Meatballs (page 200), Metabolism Advantage Salad (page 175) with either Metabolism Advantage dressing (page 182), 1 or 2 fish-oil capsules, 1 cup green tea

MEAL 3: Any Metabolism Advantage Super Shake (page 172), 1 or 2 fish-oil capsules, ½ teaspoon creatine

MEAL 4: Striped Bass with Artichoke and Asparagus (page 198), 1 or 2 fish-oil capsules, 1 cup green tea

MEAL 5: Snack or Bar (page 202), 1 cup green tea

Shopping List

DRY GOODS

- ❏ 1 can (14 ounces) artichoke hearts
- ❏ 1 can (8 ounces) juice-packed pineapple chunks
- ❏ 3 cans (15½ ounces each) chickpeas
- ❏ 1 can (15½ ounces) kidney beans
- ❏ 1 can (15½ ounces) sliced black olives, preferably Greek

PRODUCE

- ❏ 1 Roma tomato
- ❏ 10 tomatoes
- ❏ 3 oranges
- ❏ 6 onions
- ❏ 11 medium scallions
- ❏ 1 pound broccoli
- ❏ 2 ounces mushrooms
- ❏ 2 green apples
- ❏ 1 head iceberg lettuce
- ❏ 1 can (5 ounces) water chestnuts
- ❏ 4–5 ounces bean sprouts
- ❏ 2 medium acorn squash
- ❏ 20 large asparagus spears, plus 1 pound
- ❏ 1 green bell pepper
- ❏ 1 red bell pepper
- ❏ 1 yellow bell pepper
- ❏ 2 heads garlic
- ❏ 4 large lemons
- ❏ 2 limes
- ❏ 5 ounces fresh or frozen green beans
- ❏ 5 avocados
- ❏ 5 snow peas
- ❏ 1 pound baby carrots
- ❏ 2 or 3 large carrots
- ❏ 1 red onion
- ❏ 2 small jalapeños or 2 cans (4 ounces) sliced jalapeños
- ❏ ¾ pound fresh spinach
- ❏ 2 large cucumbers
- ❏ 2 bunches fresh parsley
- ❏ 1 bunch fresh cilantro
- ❏ 6-inch piece fresh ginger
- ❏ 1 bunch fresh mint

REFRIGERATED ITEMS

- ❏ 2 large containers (32 ounces each) pasteurized egg whites
- ❏ 1 dozen omega-3 eggs
- ❏ 2 cups shredded Colby cheese
- ❏ 1 container (8 ounces) low-fat, lactose-free plain yogurt
- ❏ 4 ounces mozzarella cheese, sliced
- ❏ 4 ounces Parmesan cheese
- ❏ 4 ounces feta cheese

MEAT AND FISH

- ❏ 12 ounces boneless, skinless chicken breasts
- ❏ 2⅓ pounds extra-lean (96%) ground beef
- ❏ 4 ounces turkey ham
- ❏ 2 ounces lean turkey sausage or turkey bacon
- ❏ 2 pounds salmon fillets
- ❏ 1½ pounds sea scallops
- ❏ 1½ pounds striped bass fillets, with skin

CONDIMENTS, SPICES, MISCELLANEOUS

- ❏ Ingredients for 12 Super Shakes (page 172)
- ❏ 1 container (32 ounces; approximately 10 servings) recovery drink
- ❏ Ingredients for 1 Snack or Bar (page 202)
- ❏ Fish-oil capsules
- ❏ Three servings of 10 percent meal
- ❏ Tahini
- ❏ Spicy hot V8
- ❏ 1 packet chili seasoning
- ❏ Dried thyme
- ❏ Cayenne pepper

CHECK QUANTITY AND FRESHNESS OF:

- ❏ Mixed beans (need 1 cup total)
- ❏ Shredded Cheddar cheese (need ¼ cup)
- ❏ Salsa
- ❏ Green tea

Goal Setting

Look back over your results from the previous week. If you got all your workouts in, give yourself a pat on the back. If not, list three ways you can increase your success in the coming week.

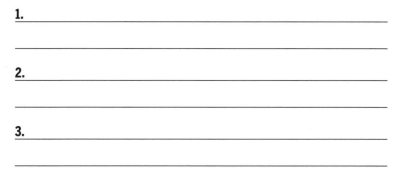

1. _____

_____

2. _____

_____

3. _____

_____

Week 2

■ **DAY 8: MONDAY**

Meal Plan

MEAL 1: The Big Omelet (page 171), 1 green apple, 1 or 2 fish-oil capsules, 1 cup green tea

MEAL 2: Any Metabolism Advantage Super Shake (page 172), 1 or 2 fish-oil capsules, ½ teaspoon creatine

MEAL 3: Teriyaki Lettuce Wrap (page 184), roasted red peppers, 1 or 2 fish-oil capsules

MEAL 4: Any Metabolism Advantage Super Shake (page 172), 1 or 2 fish-oil capsules, ½ teaspoon creatine

MEAL 5 (DURING WORKOUT): ½ recovery drink

MEAL 6 (POSTWORKOUT AT 7 PM): ½ recovery drink

MEAL 7: Citrus Chicken–Stuffed Acorn Squash (page 185), Toasted Quinoa Salad (page 176), 1 or 2 fish-oil capsules, 1 cup green tea

Lower-Body Strengthening Workout (page 99)

5-MINUTE CARDIOVASCULAR WARMUP:	Bicycling, walking, rowing, or stairclimbing
BARBELL SQUAT: 2 sets of 5–7 reps	Set 1: ___ lb ___ reps Set 2: ___ lb ___ reps
OVERHEAD BARBELL SQUAT: 2 sets of 5–7 reps	Set 1: ___ lb ___ reps Set 2: ___ lb ___ reps
BARBELL DEADLIFT: 3 sets of 5–7 reps	Set 1: ___ lb ___ reps Set 2: ___ lb ___ reps Set 3: ___ lb ___ reps
DUMBBELL WALKING LUNGE: 2 sets of 5–7 reps with each leg	Set 1: ___ lb ___ reps per leg Set 2: ___ lb ___ reps per leg
SINGLE-LEG SWISS BALL LEG CURL: 2 sets of 5–7 reps with each leg	Set 1 (right leg): ___ reps Set 1 (left leg): ___ reps Set 2 (right leg): ___ reps Set 2 (left leg): ___ reps
STEPUP: 2 sets of 5–7 reps on each side	Set 1: ___ lb ___ reps per side Set 2: ___ lb ___ reps per side
5-MINUTE CARDIOVASCULAR COOLDOWN:	Bicycling, walking, rowing, or stairclimbing

DAY 9: TUESDAY

Meal Plan

MEAL 1: Greek Omelet (page 167), 1 orange, 1 or 2 fish-oil capsules, 1 cup green tea

MEAL 2: Any Metabolism Advantage Super Shake (page 172), 1 or 2 fish-oil capsules, $\frac{1}{2}$ teaspoon creatine

MEAL 3: Roasted chicken breast, Hummus (page 179) with celery sticks, 1 or 2 fish-oil capsules

MEAL 4: Any Metabolism Advantage Super Shake (page 172), 1 or 2 fish-oil capsules, $\frac{1}{2}$ teaspoon creatine

MEAL 5 (DURING WORKOUT): $\frac{1}{2}$ recovery drink

MEAL 6 (POSTWORKOUT): $\frac{1}{2}$ recovery drink

MEAL 7: Rosemary Salmon and Asparagus on the Grill (page 192), Toasted Quinoa Salad (page 176), 1 or 2 fish-oil capsules, 1 cup green tea

Interval Workout #1

5-MINUTE LOW-INTENSITY WARMUP

INTERVALS: 30 seconds at high intensity, 90 seconds at low intensity	Perform 7 total intervals

5-MINUTE LOW-INTENSITY COOLDOWN

■ DAY 10: WEDNESDAY

Meal Plan

MEAL 1: Spinach and Cheese Omelet (page 168), 1 green apple, 1 or 2 fish-oil capsules, 1 cup green tea

MEAL 2: Any Metabolism Advantage Super Shake (page 172), 1 or 2 fish-oil capsules, ½ teaspoon creatine

MEAL 3: Leftover Rosemary Salmon from previous day, crumbled on Metabolism Advantage Salad (page 175) with either Metabolism Advantage dressing (page 182), 1 or 2 fish-oil capsules

MEAL 4: Any Metabolism Advantage Super Shake (page 172), 1 or 2 fish-oil capsules, ½ teaspoon creatine

MEAL 5 (DURING WORKOUT): ½ recovery drink

MEAL 6 (POSTWORKOUT): ½ recovery drink

MEAL 7: Greek Burger, Foreman-Style (page 194), Mixed-Bean Salad (page 180), Toasted Quinoa Salad (page 176), 1 or 2 fish-oil capsules, 1 cup green tea

Upper-Body Strengthening Workout (page 105)

5-MINUTE CARDIOVASCULAR WARMUP:	Bicycling, walking, rowing, or stairclimbing
BENT-OVER BARBELL ROW: 3 sets of 5–7 reps (2 sets with overhand grip, 1 set with underhand grip)	Set 1 (overhand grip): ___ lb ___ reps Set 2 (overhand grip): ___ lb ___ reps Set 3 (underhand grip): ___ lb ___ reps
FLAT BARBELL BENCH PRESS: 3 sets of 5–7 reps (1 set with medium grip, 1 set with wide grip, 1 set with narrow grip)	Set 1 (medium grip): ___ lb ___ reps Set 2 (wide grip): ___ lb ___ reps Set 3 (narrow grip): ___ lb ___ reps
PULLUP: 2 sets of 5–7 reps	Set 1: ___ reps Set 2: ___ reps
BARBELL OVERHEAD PRESS: 2 sets of 5–7 reps	Set 1: ___ lb ___ reps Set 2: ___ lb ___ reps
SINGLE-ARM BARBELL BICEPS CURL: 2 sets of 5–7 reps with each arm	Set 1 (right arm): ___ reps Set 1 (left arm): ___ reps Set 2 (right arm): ___ reps Set 2 (left arm): ___ reps
DIP: 2 sets of 5–7 reps	Set 1: ___ reps Set 2: ___ reps
5-MINUTE CARDIOVASCULAR COOLDOWN:	Bicycling, walking, rowing, or stairclimbing

■ DAY 11: THURSDAY

Meal Plan

MEAL 1: Denver Omelet (page 170), 1 orange, 1 or 2 fish-oil capsules, 1 cup green tea

MEAL 2: Any Metabolism Advantage Super Shake (page 172), 1 or 2 fish-oil capsules, ½ teaspoon creatine

MEAL 3: 5-ounce roasted salmon fillet, Mediterranean Salad (page 176), 1 or 2 fish-oil capsules

MEAL 4: Any Metabolism Advantage Super Shake (page 172), 1 or 2 fish-oil capsules, ½ teaspoon creatine

MEAL 5 (DURING WORKOUT): ½ recovery drink

MEAL 6 (POSTWORKOUT): ½ recovery drink

MEAL 7: Almond-Crusted Sea Scallops with Tomato-Onion Gratin (page 196), Carrot Salad (page 178), 1 or 2 fish-oil capsules, 1 cup green tea

Interval Workout #2

5-MINUTE LOW-INTENSITY WARMUP

INTERVALS: Perform 7 total intervals
60 seconds at high intensity,
60 seconds at low intensity

5-MINUTE LOW-INTENSITY COOLDOWN

■ DAY 12: FRIDAY

Meal Plan

MEAL 1: Asian Scrambled Eggs (page 168), 1 orange, 1 or 2 fish-oil capsules, 1 cup green tea

MEAL 2: Any Metabolism Advantage Super Shake (page 172), 1 or 2 fish-oil capsules, ½ teaspoon creatine

MEAL 3: Roasted chicken breast, Metabolism Advantage Tabbouleh (page 181), 1 or 2 fish-oil capsules

MEAL 4: Any Metabolism Advantage Super Shake (page 172), 1 or 2 fish-oil capsules, ½ teaspoon creatine

MEAL 5 (DURING WORKOUT): ½ recovery drink

MEAL 6 (POSTWORKOUT): ½ recovery drink

MEAL 7: Chili in a Flash (page 200), Guacamole (page 180), 1 or 2 fish-oil capsules, 1 cup green tea

Total-Body Strengthening Workout (page 111)

5-MINUTE CARDIOVASCULAR WARMUP:	Bicycling, walking, rowing, or stairclimbing
PUSHUP ON SWISS BALL: 2 sets of 8–10 reps	Set 1: ___ reps Set 2: ___ reps
SUITCASE DEADLIFT: 3 sets of 8–10 reps on each side	Set 1 (right side): ___ reps Set 1 (left side): ___ reps Set 2 (right side): ___ reps Set 2 (left side): ___ reps Set 3 (right side): ___ reps Set 3 (left side): ___ reps
BARBELL CLEANS: 3 sets of 8–10 reps	Set 1: ___ lb ___ reps Set 2: ___ lb ___ reps Set 3: ___ lb ___ reps
DUMBBELL OVERHEAD WALKING LUNGES: 2 sets of 8–10 reps per leg	Set 1: ___ lb ___ reps per leg Set 2: ___ lb ___ reps per leg
BRIDGE: 2 sets of 30 seconds each	Set 1: ___ Set 2: ___
SIDE BRIDGE: 2 sets of 30 seconds on each side	Set 1 (right side): ___ Set 1 (left side): ___ Set 2 (right side): ___ Set 2 (left side): ___
5-MINUTE CARDIOVASCULAR COOLDOWN:	Bicycling, walking, rowing, or stairclimbing

■ DAY 13: SATURDAY (ASSUMING AM WORKOUT)

Meal Plan

MEAL 1: (during workout): ½ recovery drink

MEAL 2: (Postworkout): ½ recovery drink

MEAL 3: Mexican Frittata (page 170), ½ avocado or Guacamole (page 180), 1 or 2 fish-oil capsules, 1 cup green tea

MEAL 4: Any Metabolism Advantage Super Shake (page 172), 1 or 2 fish-oil capsules, ½ teaspoon creatine

MEAL 5: Quick Quinoa and Chicken (page 186), Mixed-Bean Salad (page 180), 1 or 2 fish-oil capsules

MEAL 6: 10 percent meal, 1 or 2 fish-oil capsules, 1 cup green tea

MEAL 7: Any Metabolism Advantage Super Shake (page 172), 1 or 2 fish-oil capsules, ½ teaspoon creatine

Interval Workout #3

5-MINUTE LOW-INTENSITY WARMUP

INTERVALS: 90 seconds at high intensity, 180 seconds at low intensity	Perform 4 total intervals

5-MINUTE LOW-INTENSITY COOLDOWN

■ DAY 14: SUNDAY (ASSUMING NO WORKOUT)

Meal Plan

MEAL 1: 10 percent meal, 1 or 2 fish-oil capsules, 1 cup green tea

MEAL 2: Extra-Lean Beef Meatballs (page 200), Metabolism Advantage Salad (page 175) with either Metabolism Advantage dressing (page 182), 1 or 2 fish-oil capsules, 1 cup green tea

MEAL 3: Any Metabolism Advantage Super Shake (page 172), 1 or 2 fish-oil capsules, ½ teaspoon creatine

MEAL 4: Striped Bass with Artichoke and Asparagus (page 198), 1 or 2 fish-oil capsules, 1 cup green tea

MEAL 5: Either of the Snacks and Bars (page 202), 1 cup green tea

Shopping List

DRY GOODS

- ❏ 3 cans (15½ ounces each) mixed beans (kidney beans, black beans, or chickpeas; canned), plus 3 cans (15½ ounces each) chickpeas
- ❏ 1 can (8 ounces) juice-packed pineapple chunks
- ❏ 3 cans (14 ounces each) water-packed chunk light tuna
- ❏ 1 can (15½ ounces) sliced black olives, preferably Greek
- ❏ Black mustard seed

PRODUCE

- ❏ 3 oranges
- ❏ 1 green apple
- ❏ ¼ pint strawberries
- ❏ 1 medium banana
- ❏ 1 large kiwifruit
- ❏ 3 large lemons
- ❏ 2 limes
- ❏ 9 tomatoes
- ❏ 1 Roma tomato
- ❏ 4 ounces fresh or frozen green beans
- ❏ 1 pound broccoli
- ❏ 4 onions
- ❏ 4 scallions
- ❏ 1 bunch fresh basil
- ❏ 2 pounds fresh spinach
- ❏ 2 or 3 shallots
- ❏ 2 ounces mushrooms
- ❏ 2 heads garlic
- ❏ 7 avocados
- ❏ 1 pound baby carrots
- ❏ 2 or 3 large carrots
- ❏ 1 bunch fresh cilantro
- ❏ 1 bunch fresh mint
- ❏ 1 red onion
- ❏ 2 small jalapeños or 2 cans (4 ounces each) sliced jalapeños
- ❏ 3 green bell peppers
- ❏ 1 red bell pepper
- ❏ 1 bunch celery
- ❏ 2-inch piece fresh ginger

REFRIGERATED ITEMS

- ❏ 2 large containers (32 ounces each) pasteurized egg whites
- ❏ 1 dozen omega-3 eggs
- ❏ 4 ounces feta cheese
- ❏ 1 container (8 ounces) low-fat, lactose-free plain yogurt
- ❏ 1 container (8 ounces) low-fat cottage cheese

MEATS AND FISH

- ❏ 2⅓ pounds extra-lean (96%) ground beef
- ❏ 8 ounces turkey ham
- ❏ 8 ounces turkey sausage or 6 ounces turkey sausage and 2 ounces turkey bacon

❏ 1½ pounds boneless, skinless chicken breasts
❏ 1 pound, 10 ounces salmon fillets

❏ 1½ pounds striped bass fillets, with skin

CONDIMENTS, SPICES, MISCELLANEOUS

❏ Ingredients for 13 Metabolism Advantage Super Shakes (page 172) of your choice

❏ 1 container (32 ounces; approximately 10 servings) recovery drink
❏ Ingredients for 1 Snack or Bar

CHECK QUANTITIES AND FRESHNESS OF:

❏ Butter, coconut oil, or Smart Balance spread (need 4 tablespoons)
❏ Mixed nuts (walnuts, almonds, pecans, cashews; need enough for 1 cup, plus 2 tablespoons pecan meal and ³⁄₈ cup walnuts)
❏ Quinoa
❏ Flaxseed
❏ Fish-oil capsules

❏ Salsa (need ¼ cup)
❏ White cooking wine (need ½ cup)
❏ Oat bran
❏ Wheat bran
❏ Green tea
❏ Parsley
❏ Shredded Colby cheese (need ½ cup)
❏ Shredded Cheddar cheese (need ¼ cup)

Goal Setting

Look back over your results from the previous week. If you got all your workouts in, give yourself a pat on the back. If not, list three ways you can increase your success in the coming week.

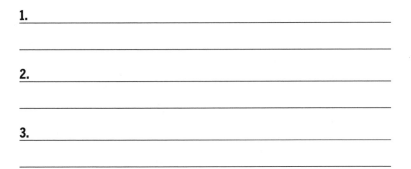

1. _____

_____

2. _____

_____

3. _____

_____

Week 3

■ **DAY 15: MONDAY**

Meal Plan

MEAL 1: Greek Omelet (page 167), 1 orange, 1 or 2 fish-oil capsules, 1 cup green tea

MEAL 2: Any Metabolism Advantage Super Shake (page 172), 1 or 2 fish-oil capsules, ½ teaspoon creatine

MEAL 3: Leftover Striped Bass from previous day, crumbled on Metabolism Advantage Salad (page 175) with either Metabolism Advantage dressing (page 182), 1 or 2 fish-oil capsules

MEAL 4: Any Metabolism Advantage Super Shake (page 172), 1 or 2 fish-oil capsules, ½ teaspoon creatine

MEAL 5 (DURING WORKOUT): ½ recovery drink

MEAL 6 (POSTWORKOUT): ½ recovery drink

MEAL 7: Pecan-Crusted Salmon (page 194), Toasted Quinoa Salad (page 176), Fruit Salad (page 178), 1 or 2 fish-oil capsules, 1 cup green tea

Lower-Body Strengthening Workout (page 99)

5-MINUTE CARDIOVASCULAR WARMUP:	Bicycling, walking, rowing, or stairclimbing
BARBELL SQUAT: 2 sets of 5–7 reps	Set 1: ___ lb ___ reps Set 2: ___ lb ___ reps
OVERHEAD BARBELL SQUAT: 2 sets of 5–7 reps	Set 1: ___ lb ___ reps Set 2: ___ lb ___ reps
BARBELL DEADLIFT: 3 sets of 5–7 reps	Set 1: ___ lb ___ reps Set 2: ___ lb ___ reps Set 3: ___ lb ___ reps
DUMBBELL WALKING LUNGE: 2 sets of 5–7 reps with each leg	Set 1: ___ lb ___ reps per leg Set 2: ___ lb ___ reps per leg
SINGLE-LEG SWISS BALL LEG CURL: 2 sets of 5–7 reps with each leg	Set 1 (right leg): ___ reps Set 1 (left leg): ___ reps Set 2 (right leg): ___ reps Set 2 (left leg): ___ reps
STEPUP: 2 sets of 5–7 reps on each side	Set 1: ___ lb ___ reps per side Set 2: ___ lb ___ reps per side
5-MINUTE CARDIOVASCULAR COOLDOWN:	Bicycling, walking, rowing, or stairclimbing

■ DAY 16: TUESDAY

Meal Plan

MEAL 1: Denver Omelet (page 170), $\frac{1}{2}$ avocado, 1 or 2 fish-oil capsules, 1 cup green tea

MEAL 2: Any Metabolism Advantage Super Shake (page 172), 1 or 2 fish-oil capsules, $\frac{1}{2}$ teaspoon creatine

MEAL 3: Leftover Pecan-Crusted Salmon from previous day crumbled on Metabolism Advantage Salad (page 175) with either Metabolism Advantage dressing (page 182), 1 or 2 fish-oil capsules

MEAL 4: Any Metabolism Advantage Super Shake (page 172), 1 or 2 fish-oil capsules, $\frac{1}{2}$ teaspoon creatine

MEAL 5 (DURING WORKOUT): $\frac{1}{2}$ recovery drink

MEAL 6 (POSTWORKOUT): $\frac{1}{2}$ recovery drink

MEAL 7: Meta Meat Loaf (page 201), Grilled Peppers and Tomatoes (page 177), 1 or 2 fish-oil capsules, 1 cup green tea

Interval Workout #1

5-MINUTE LOW-INTENSITY WARMUP

INTERVALS: 30 seconds at high intensity, 90 seconds at low intensity	Perform 7 total intervals

5-MINUTE LOW-INTENSITY COOLDOWN

DAY 17: WEDNESDAY

Meal Plan

MEAL 1: The Big Omelet (page 171), 1 orange, 1 or 2 fish-oil capsules, 1 cup green tea

MEAL 2: Any Metabolism Advantage Super Shake (page 172), 1 or 2 fish-oil capsules, ½ teaspoon creatine

MEAL 3: Leftover Meta Meat Loaf from previous day, Hummus (page 179) with celery sticks, 1 or 2 fish-oil capsules

MEAL 4: Any Metabolism Advantage Super Shake (page 172), 1 or 2 fish-oil capsules, 1½ teaspoon creatine

MEAL 5 (DURING WORKOUT): ½ recovery drink

MEAL 6 (POSTWORKOUT): ½ recovery drink

MEAL 7: Salmon in Basil Cream Sauce (page 193), Metabolism Advantage Salad (page 175) with either Metabolism Advantage dressing (page 182), Toasted Quinoa Salad (page 176), 1 or 2 fish-oil capsules, 1 cup green tea

Upper-Body Strengthening Workout (page 105)

5-MINUTE CARDIOVASCULAR WARMUP:	Bicycling, walking, rowing, or stairclimbing
BENT-OVER BARBELL ROW: 3 sets of 5–7 reps (2 sets with overhand grip, 1 set with underhand grip)	Set 1 (overhand grip): ___ lb ___ reps Set 2 (overhand grip): ___ lb ___ reps Set 3 (underhand grip): ___ lb ___ reps
FLAT BARBELL BENCH PRESS: 3 sets of 5–7 reps (1 set with medium grip, 1 set with wide grip, 1 set with narrow grip)	Set 1 (medium grip): ___ lb ___ reps Set 2 (wide grip): ___ lb ___ reps Set 3 (narrow grip): ___ lb ___ reps
PULLUP: 2 sets of 5–7 reps	Set 1: ___ reps Set 2: ___ reps
BARBELL OVERHEAD PRESS: 2 sets of 5–7 reps	Set 1: ___ lb ___ reps Set 2: ___ lb ___ reps
SINGLE-ARM BARBELL BICEPS CURL: 2 sets of 5–7 reps with each arm	Set 1 (right arm): ___ reps Set 1 (left arm): ___ reps Set 2 (right arm): ___ reps Set 2 (left arm): ___ reps
DIP: 2 sets of 5–7 reps	Set 1: ___ reps Set 2: ___ reps
5-MINUTE CARDIOVASCULAR COOLDOWN:	Bicycling, walking, rowing, or stairclimbing

DAY 18: THURSDAY

Meal Plan

MEAL 1: Scrambled Eggs and Greens (page 169), 1 green apple, 1 or 2 fish-oil capsules, 1 cup green tea

MEAL 2: Any Metabolism Advantage Super Shake (page 172), 1 or 2 fish-oil capsules, ½ teaspoon creatine

MEAL 3: Leftover Basil Salmon from previous day, crumbled onto Metabolism Advantage Salad (page 175) with either Metabolism Advantage dressing (page 182), 1 or 2 fish-oil capsules

MEAL 4: Any Metabolism Advantage Super Shake (page 172), 1 or 2 fish-oil capsules, ½ teaspoon creatine

MEAL 5 (DURING WORKOUT): ½ recovery drink

MEAL 6 (POSTWORKOUT): ½ recovery drink

MEAL 7: Greek Burger (page 194), Toasted Quinoa Salad (page 176), 1 or 2 fish-oil capsules, 1 cup green tea

Interval Workout #2

5-MINUTE LOW-INTENSITY WARMUP

INTERVALS: 60 seconds at high intensity, 60 seconds at low intensity	Perform 7 total intervals

5-MINUTE LOW-INTENSITY COOLDOWN

DAY 19: FRIDAY

Meal Plan

MEAL 1: Spinach and Cheese Omelet (page 168), 1 orange, 1 or 2 fish-oil capsules, 1 cup green tea

MEAL 2: Any Metabolism Advantage Super Shake (page 172), 1 or 2 fish-oil capsules, $\frac{1}{2}$ teaspoon creatine

MEAL 3: Roasted chicken breast, Metabolism Advantage Salad (page 175) with either Metabolism Advantage dressing (page 182), 1 or 2 fish-oil capsules

MEAL 4: Any Metabolism Advantage Super Shake (page 172), 1 or 2 fish-oil capsules, $\frac{1}{2}$ teaspoon creatine

MEAL 5 (DURING WORKOUT): $\frac{1}{2}$ recovery drink

MEAL 6 (POSTWORKOUT): $\frac{1}{2}$ recovery drink

MEAL 7: Tuna Burger (page 195), Carrot Salad (page 178), 1 or 2 fish-oil capsules, 1 cup green tea

Total-Body Strengthening Workout (page 111)

5-MINUTE CARDIOVASCULAR WARMUP:	Bicycling, walking, rowing, or stairclimbing
PUSHUP ON SWISS BALL: 2 sets of 8–10 reps	Set 1: ___ reps Set 2: ___ reps
SUITCASE DEADLIFT: 3 sets of 8–10 reps on each side	Set 1 (right side): ___ reps Set 1 (left side): ___ reps Set 2 (right side): ___ reps Set 2 (left side): ___ reps Set 3 (right side): ___ reps Set 3 (left side): ___ reps
BARBELL CLEAN: 3 sets of 8–10 reps	Set 1: ___ lb ___ reps Set 2: ___ lb ___ reps Set 3: ___ lb ___ reps
DUMBBELL OVERHEAD WALKING LUNGE: 2 sets of 8–10 reps with each leg	Set 1: ___ lb ___ reps per leg Set 2: ___ lb ___ reps per leg
BRIDGE: 2 sets of 30 seconds each	Set 1: ___ Set 2: ___
SIDE BRIDGE: 2 sets of 30 seconds on each side	Set 1 (right side): ___ Set 1 (left side): ___ Set 2 (right side): ___ Set 2 (left side): ___
5-MINUTE CARDIOVASCULAR COOLDOWN:	Bicycling, walking, rowing, or stairclimbing

DAY 20: SATURDAY (ASSUMING AM WORKOUT)

Meal Plan

MEAL 1 (DURING WORKOUT): $\frac{1}{2}$ recovery drink

MEAL 2 (POSTWORKOUT): $\frac{1}{2}$ recovery drink

MEAL 3: Mexican Frittata (page 170), $\frac{1}{2}$ avocado or Guacamole (page 180), 1 or 2 fish-oil capsules, 1 cup green tea

MEAL 4: Any Metabolism Advantage Super Shake (page 172), 1 or 2 fish-oil capsules, $\frac{1}{2}$ teaspoon creatine

MEAL 5: Quick Quinoa and Chicken (page 186), Mixed-Bean Salad (page 180), 1 or 2 fish-oil capsules

MEAL 6: 10 percent meal, 1 or 2 fish-oil capsules, 1 cup green tea

MEAL 7: Any Metabolism Advantage Super Shake (page 172), 1 or 2 fish-oil capsules, $\frac{1}{2}$ teaspoon creatine

Interval Workout #3

5-MINUTE LOW-INTENSITY WARMUP

INTERVALS: 90 seconds at high intensity, 180 seconds at low intensity	Perform 4 total intervals

5-MINUTE LOW-INTENSITY COOLDOWN

DAY 21: SUNDAY (ASSUMING NO WORKOUT)

Meal Plan

MEAL 1: 10 percent meal, 1 or 2 fish-oil capsules, 1 cup green tea

MEAL 2: Extra-Lean Beef Meatballs (page 200), Metabolism Advantage Salad (page 175) with either Metabolism Advantage dressing (page 182), 1 or 2 fish-oil capsules, 1 cup green tea

MEAL 3: Any Metabolism Advantage Super Shake (page 172), 1 or 2 fish-oil capsules, $\frac{1}{2}$ teaspoon creatine

MEAL 4: Striped Bass with Artichoke and Asparagus (page 198), 1 or 2 fish-oil capsules, 1 cup green tea

MEAL 5: Snack or Bar (page 202), 1 cup green tea

Shopping List

DRY GOODS

- 3 cans (15½ ounces) mixed beans (kidney beans, black beans, or chickpeas) plus 1 can (15½ ounces) kidney beans
- 1 can (5 ounces) water chestnuts
- 1 can (8 ounces) roasted red peppers
- 1 can (8 ounces) juice-packed pineapple chunks
- 1 can (15½ ounces) sliced black olives, preferably Greek)

PRODUCE

- 1 pound (20 large spears) asparagus
- 1 pound fresh spinach
- 1 head iceberg lettuce
- 8 tomatoes
- 1 head cabbage
- 1 Roma tomato
- 2 pounds broccoli
- 3 avocados
- 1 pound baby carrots
- 3 or 4 large carrots
- 1 large cucumber
- 8 ounces fresh mushrooms
- 3 medium scallions
- 5 onions
- 1 red onion
- 1 small jalapeño or 1 can (4 ounces) sliced jalapeños
- 1-inch piece fresh ginger
- 3 limes
- 5 snow peas
- 4–5 ounces bean sprouts
- 3 green bell peppers
- 1 red bell pepper
- 1 yellow bell pepper
- 5 ounces fresh or frozen green beans
- 4 oranges
- ¼ pint strawberries
- 1 medium banana
- 1 large kiwifruit
- 3 lemons
- 1 or 2 heads garlic
- 1 bunch fresh rosemary
- 1 bunch fresh cilantro
- 1 bunch fresh mint

REFRIGERATED ITEMS

- 2 large containers (32 ounces each) pasteurized egg whites
- 1 dozen omega-3 eggs
- 2 ounces feta cheese
- 1 container (8 ounces) low-fat, lactose-free plain yogurt

MEATS AND FISH

- 1 pound, 10 ounces salmon fillets
- 1 can (14¾ ounces) salmon
- 1½ pounds striped bass fillets, with skin
- 6 ounces lean turkey sausage
- 2 ounces turkey sausage or turkey bacon
- 4 ounces turkey ham

❏ 1½ pounds extra-lean (96%) ground beef

❏ 4½ pounds boneless, skinless chicken breasts

CONDIMENTS, SPICES, MISCELLANEOUS

❏ Ingredients for 13 Super Shakes (page 172) of your choice
❏ 1 container (32 ounces; approximately 10 servings) recovery drink

❏ Ingredients for 2 servings 10 percent meal
❏ 1 packet chili powder
❏ Turmeric
❏ Chicken bouillon

CHECK QUANTITIES AND FRESHNESS OF:

❏ Mixed nuts (walnuts, almonds, pecans, cashews; need ⅔ cup mixed plus ¼ cup walnuts, 2 tablespoons pecan meal, and ½ cup cashews)
❏ Quinoa (need ½ cup)
❏ Flaxseed (need ¼ cup meal and ⅛ cup ground)
❏ Fish-oil capsules
❏ Oat bran (need ¼ cup)
❏ Wheat bran (need ⅛ cup)
❏ Green tea
❏ Spicy Hot V-8 (need 1 cup)

❏ Peanut sauce
❏ Olive oil
❏ Butter, coconut oil, or Smart Balance spread
❏ Shredded Colby cheese (need ½ cup)
❏ Shredded Cheddar cheese (need ¼ cup)
❏ Fat-free American cheese (need 2 slices)
❏ Salsa (need ¼ cup)
❏ Dry white wine (need 2 tablespoons)
❏ Cooking wine (need 2 tablespoons)

Goal Setting

Look back over your results from the previous week. If you got all your workouts in, give yourself a pat on the back. If not, list three ways you can increase your success in the coming week.

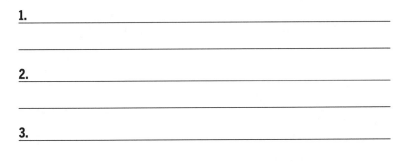

1. _____

_____

2. _____

_____

3. _____

_____

Week 4

■ DAY 22: MONDAY

Meal Plan

MEAL 1: Asian Scrambled Eggs (page 168), 1 orange, 1 or 2 fish-oil capsules, 1 cup green tea

MEAL 2: Any Metabolism Advantage Super Shake (page 172), 1 or 2 fish-oil capsules, ½ teaspoon creatine

MEAL 3: Roasted chicken breast, roasted red peppers, 1 or 2 fish-oil capsules

MEAL 4: Any Metabolism Advantage Super Shake (page 172), 1 or 2 fish-oil capsules, ½ teaspoon creatine

MEAL 5 (DURING WORKOUT): ½ recovery drink

MEAL 6 (POSTWORKOUT): ½ recovery drink

MEAL 7: Rosemary Salmon and Asparagus on the Grill (page 192), Grilled Peppers and Tomatoes (page 177), Fruit Salad (page 178), 1 or 2 fish-oil capsules, 1 cup green tea

Lower-Body Strengthening Workout (page 99)

5-MINUTE CARDIOVASCULAR WARMUP:	Bicycling, walking, rowing, or stairclimbing
BARBELL SQUAT: 2 sets of 5–7 reps	Set 1: ___ lb ___ reps Set 2: ___ lb ___ reps
OVERHEAD BARBELL SQUAT: 2 sets of 5–7 reps	Set 1: ___ lb ___ reps Set 2: ___ lb ___ reps
BARBELL DEADLIFT: 3 sets of 5–7 reps	Set 1: ___ lb ___ reps Set 2: ___ lb ___ reps Set 3: ___ lb ___ reps
DUMBBELL WALKING LUNGE: 2 sets of 5–7 reps with each leg	Set 1: ___ lb ___ reps per leg Set 2: ___ lb ___ reps per leg
SINGLE-LEG SWISS BALL LEG CURL: 2 sets of 5–7 reps with each leg	Set 1 (right leg): ___ reps Set 1 (left leg): ___ reps Set 2 (right leg): ___ reps Set 2 (left leg): ___ reps
STEPUP: 2 sets of 5–7 reps on each side	Set 1: ___ lb ___ reps per side Set 2: ___ lb ___ reps per side
5-MINUTE CARDIOVASCULAR COOLDOWN:	Bicycling, walking, rowing, or stairclimbing

■ DAY 23: TUESDAY

Meal Plan

MEAL 1: The Big Omelet (page 171), 1 orange, 1 or 2 fish-oil capsules, 1 cup green tea

MEAL 2: Any Metabolism Advantage Super Shake (page 172), 1 or 2 fish-oil capsules, ½ teaspoon creatine

MEAL 3: Leftover Rosemary Salmon from previous day, crumbled on Metabolism Advantage Salad (page 175) with either Metabolism Advantage dressing (page 182), 1 or 2 fish-oil capsules

MEAL 4: Any Metabolism Advantage Super Shake (page 172), 1 or 2 fish-oil capsules, ½ teaspoon creatine

MEAL 5 (DURING WORKOUT): ½ recovery drink

MEAL 6 (POSTWORKOUT): ½ recovery drink

MEAL 7: Chili in a Flash (page 200), Toasted Quinoa Salad (page 176), 1 or 2 fish-oil capsules, 1 cup green tea

Interval Workout #1

5-MINUTE LOW-INTENSITY WARMUP

INTERVALS: 30 seconds at high intensity, 90 seconds at low intensity	Perform 7 total intervals

5-MINUTE LOW-INTENSITY COOLDOWN

DAY 24: WEDNESDAY

MEAL 1: Denver Omelet (page 170), 1 orange, 1 or 2 fish-oil capsules, 1 cup green tea

MEAL 2: Any Metabolism Advantage Super Shake (page 172), 1 or 2 fish-oil capsules, 1½ teaspoon creatine

MEAL 3: Roasted chicken breast, Metabolism Advantage Salad (page 175) with either Metabolism Advantage dressing (page 182), 1 or 2 fish-oil capsules

MEAL 4: Any Metabolism Advantage Super Shake (page 172), 1 or 2 fish-oil capsules, ½ teaspoon creatine

MEAL 5 (DURING WORKOUT): ½ recovery drink

MEAL 6 (POSTWORKOUT): ½ recovery drink

MEAL 7: Salmon Burger Stroganoff (page 191), Mixed-Bean Salad (page 180), Toasted Quinoa Salad (page 176), 1 or 2 fish-oil capsules, 1 cup green tea

Upper-Body Strengthening Workout (page 105)

5-MINUTE CARDIOVASCULAR WARMUP:	Bicycling, walking, rowing, or stairclimbing
BENT-OVER BARBELL ROW: 3 sets of 5–7 reps (2 sets with overhand grip, 1 set with underhand grip)	Set 1 (overhand grip): ___ lb ___ reps Set 2 (overhand grip): ___ lb ___ reps Set 3 (underhand grip): ___ lb ___ reps
FLAT BARBELL BENCH PRESS: 3 sets of 5–7 reps (1 set with medium grip, 1 set with wide grip, 1 set with narrow grip)	Set 1 (medium grip): ___ lb ___ reps Set 2 (wide grip): ___ lb ___ reps Set 3 (narrow grip): ___ lb ___ reps
PULLUP: 2 sets of 5–7 reps	Set 1: ___ reps Set 2: ___ reps
BARBELL OVERHEAD PRESS: 2 sets of 5–7 reps	Set 1: ___ lb ___ reps Set 2: ___ lb ___ reps
SINGLE-ARM BARBELL BICEPS CURL: 2 sets of 5–7 reps with each arm	Set 1 (right arm): ___ reps Set 1 (left arm): ___ reps Set 2 (right arm): ___ reps Set 2 (left arm): ___ reps
DIP: 2 sets of 5–7 reps	Set 1: ___ reps Set 2: ___ reps
5-MINUTE CARDIOVASCULAR COOLDOWN:	Bicycling, walking, rowing, or stairclimbing

DAY 25: THURSDAY

Meal Plan

MEAL 1: Scrambled Eggs and Greens (page 169), $\frac{1}{2}$ avocado,
1 or 2 fish-oil capsules, 1 cup green tea

MEAL 2: Any Metabolism Advantage Super Shake (page 172),
1 or 2 fish-oil capsules, $\frac{1}{2}$ teaspoon creatine

MEAL 3: Roasted chicken breast (page 186), Mediterranean Salad
(page 176), 1 or 2 fish-oil capsules

MEAL 4: Any Metabolism Advantage Super Shake (page 172),
1 or 2 fish-oil capsules, $\frac{1}{2}$ teaspoon creatine

MEAL 5 (DURING WORKOUT): $\frac{1}{2}$ recovery drink

MEAL 6 (POSTWORKOUT): $\frac{1}{2}$ recovery drink

MEAL 7: Thai Ground Beef (page 199), Mashed Garlic Cauliflower
(page 181), 1 or 2 fish-oil capsules, 1 cup green tea

Interval Workout #2

**5-MINUTE LOW-INTENSITY
WARMUP**

INTERVALS: Perform 7 total intervals
60 seconds at high intensity,
60 seconds at low intensity

**5-MINUTE LOW-INTENSITY
COOLDOWN**

DAY 26: FRIDAY

Meal Plan

MEAL 1: Greek Omelet (page 167), 1 orange, 1 or 2 fish-oil capsules, 1 cup green tea

MEAL 2: Any Metabolism Advantage Super Shake (page 172), 1 or 2 fish-oil capsules, ½ teaspoon creatine

MEAL 3: Teriyaki Lettuce Wrap (page 184), roasted red peppers, 1 or 2 fish-oil capsules

MEAL 4: Any Metabolism Advantage Super Shake (page 172), 1 or 2 fish-oil capsules, ½ teaspoon creatine

MEAL 5 (DURING WORKOUT): ½ recovery drink

MEAL 6 (POSTWORKOUT): ½ recovery drink

MEAL 7: Quick Quinoa and Chicken (page 186), Carrot Salad (page 178), 1 or 2 fish-oil capsules, 1 cup green tea

Total-Body Strengthening Workout (page 111)

5-MINUTE CARDIOVASCULAR WARMUP:	Bicycling, walking, rowing, or stairclimbing
PUSHUP ON SWISS BALL: 2 sets of 8–10 reps	Set 1: ___ reps Set 2: ___ reps
SUITCASE DEADLIFT: 3 sets of 8–10 reps on each side	Set 1 (right side): ___ reps Set 1 (left side): ___ reps Set 2 (right side): ___ reps Set 2 (left side): ___ reps Set 3 (right side): ___ reps Set 3 (left side): ___ reps
BARBELL CLEAN: 3 sets of 8–10 reps	Set 1: ___ lb ___ reps Set 2: ___ lb ___ reps Set 3: ___ lb ___ reps
DUMBBELL OVERHEAD WALKING LUNGE: 2 sets of 8–10 reps with each leg	Set 1: ___ lb ___ reps per leg Set 2: ___ lb ___ reps per leg
BRIDGE: 2 sets of 30 seconds each	Set 1: ___ Set 2: ___
SIDE BRIDGE: 2 sets of 30 seconds on each side	Set 1 (right side): ___ Set 1 (left side): ___ Set 2 (right side): ___ Set 2 (left side): ___
5-MINUTE CARDIOVASCULAR COOLDOWN:	Bicycling, walking, rowing, or stairclimbing

DAY 27: SATURDAY (ASSUMING AM WORKOUT)

Meal Plan

MEAL 1 (DURING WORKOUT): ½ recovery drink

MEAL 2 (POSTWORKOUT): ½ recovery drink

MEAL 3: Mexican Frittata (page 170), ½ avocado or Guacamole (page 180), 1 or 2 fish-oil capsules, 1 cup green tea

MEAL 4: Any Metabolism Advantage Super Shake (page 172), 1 or 2 fish-oil capsules, ½ teaspoon creatine

MEAL 5: Pecan-Crusted Salmon (page 194), Mixed-Bean Salad (page 180), 1 or 2 fish-oil capsules

MEAL 6: 10 percent meal, 1 or 2 fish-oil capsules, 1 cup green tea

MEAL 7: Any Metabolism Advantage Super Shake (page 172), 1 or 2 fish-oil capsules, ½ teaspoon creatine

Interval Workout #3

5-MINUTE LOW-INTENSITY WARMUP

| **INTERVALS:** | Perform 4 total intervals |
| 90 seconds at high intensity, 180 seconds at low intensity | |

5-MINUTE LOW-INTENSITY COOLDOWN

DAY 28: SUNDAY (ASSUMING NO WORKOUT)

Meal Plan

MEAL 1: 10 percent meal, 1 or 2 fish-oil capsules, 1 cup green tea

MEAL 2: Extra-Lean Beef Meatballs (page 200), Metabolism Advantage Salad (page 175) with either Metabolism Advantage dressing (page 182), 1 or 2 fish-oil capsules, 1 cup green tea

MEAL 3: Any Metabolism Advantage Super Shake (page 172), 1 or 2 fish-oil capsules, ½ teaspoon creatine

MEAL 4: Striped Bass with Artichoke and Asparagus (page 198), 1 or 2 fish-oil capsules, 1 cup green tea

MEAL 5: Snack or Bar (page 202), 1 cup green tea

Shopping List

DRY GOODS

- ❑ 1 can (14 ounces) artichoke hearts
- ❑ 1 can (15½ ounces) sliced black olives, preferably Greek
- ❑ 3 cans (15½ ounces each) mixed beans (kidney beans, black beans, chickpeas)
- ❑ 1 can (8 ounces) juice-packed pineapple chunks

PRODUCE

- ❑ 2 pounds fresh spinach
- ❑ 9 tomatoes
- ❑ 4 avocados (plus 5 more if you want to substitute homemade guacamole)
- ❑ 2½ pounds broccoli
- ❑ 1 pound baby carrots
- ❑ 2 or 3 carrots
- ❑ 4 ounces fresh mushrooms
- ❑ 4 medium onions
- ❑ 1 red onion
- ❑ 3 medium scallions
- ❑ 1 head garlic
- ❑ 2 or 3 shallots
- ❑ 2 green bell peppers
- ❑ 1 red bell pepper
- ❑ 1 large cucumber
- ❑ 5 snow peas
- ❑ 1 bunch fresh cilantro
- ❑ 1 bunch fresh mint
- ❑ 1 bunch fresh parsley
- ❑ 1 pound asparagus
- ❑ 1 bunch fresh basil
- ❑ 1 small jalapeño pepper or 1 can (4 ounces) sliced jalapeños
- ❑ 1-inch piece fresh ginger
- ❑ 1 lime
- ❑ 3 large lemons
- ❑ 5 ounces fresh or frozen green beans
- ❑ 3 oranges
- ❑ 1 green apple
- ❑ ¼ pint strawberries
- ❑ 1 medium banana
- ❑ 1 large kiwifruit

REFRIGERATED ITEMS

- ❑ 2 large containers (32 ounces each) pasteurized egg whites
- ❑ 1 dozen omega-3 eggs
- ❑ 4 ounces feta cheese
- ❑ 8 ounces low-fat cottage cheese
- ❑ 1 container (8 ounces) low-fat, lactose-free plain yogurt

MEAT AND FISH

- ❑ 3¼ pounds salmon fillets
- ❑ 1½ pounds striped bass fillets, with skin
- ❑ 1½ pounds boneless, skinless chicken breast
- ❑ 2 pounds extra-lean (96%) ground beef
- ❑ 4 ounces turkey ham
- ❑ 2 ounces turkey sausage or turkey bacon

CONDIMENTS, SPICES, MISCELLANEOUS

❏ Ingredients for Metabolism Advantage Salad dressing (page 182) of your choice

❏ Ingredients for 1 Snack or Bar (page 202) of your choice

❏ Ingredients for 13 Super Shakes (page 172) of your choice

❏ Ingredients for 4 servings of 10 percent meal

❏ 1 container (32 ounces; approximately 10 servings) recovery drink

CHECK QUANTITIES AND FRESHNESS OF:

❏ Butter, coconut oil, or Smart Balance spread

❏ Fish-oil capsules

❏ Green tea

❏ Shelled mixed nuts (walnuts, almonds, pecans, cashews; need 1 cup mixed plus 1/4 cup walnuts and 2 tablespoons pecan meal)

❏ Oat bran (need 1/2 cup)

❏ Wheat bran (need 1/4 cup)

❏ Quinoa (need 1 1/2 cups)

❏ Flaxseed (need 2 tablespoons whole or 4 tablespoons ground plus 1/4 cup ground)

❏ Fat-free American cheese (need 1 slice)

❏ Mozzarella cheese (need 1 slice)

❏ Shredded Cheddar cheese (need 1/4 cup)

❏ Celery (need 2 stalks)

❏ Dry cooking wine (need 1/3 cup)

❏ Dry white wine (need 1 1/2 tablespoons)

❏ Salsa (need 1/4 cup)

Goal Setting

Look back over your results from the previous week. If you got all your workouts in, give yourself a pat on the back. If not, list three ways you can increase your success in the coming week.

1. _____

_____

2. _____

_____

3. _____

_____

Week 5

■ DAY 29: MONDAY

Meal Plan

MEAL 1: Greek Omelet (page 167), 1 orange, 1 or 2 fish-oil capsules, 1 cup green tea

MEAL 2: Any Metabolism Advantage Super Shake (page 172), 1 or 2 fish-oil capsules, ½ teaspoon creatine

MEAL 3: 5-ounce roasted salmon fillet, Metabolism Advantage Salad (page 175) with either Metabolism Advantage dressing (page 182), 1 or 2 fish-oil capsules

MEAL 4: Any Metabolism Advantage Super Shake (page 172), 1 or 2 fish-oil capsules, ½ teaspoon creatine

MEAL 5 (DURING WORKOUT): ½ recovery drink

MEAL 6 (POSTWORKOUT): ½ recovery drink

MEAL 7: Meta Meat Loaf (page 201), Metabolism Advantage Spinach Sauté (page 175), Toasted Quinoa Salad (page 176), 1 or 2 fish-oil capsules, 1 cup green tea

Lower-Body Strengthening Workout (page 117)

5-MINUTE CARDIOVASCULAR WARMUP:	Bicycling, walking, rowing, or stairclimbing
BARBELL GOOD MORNING: 3 sets of 5–7 reps	Set 1: ___ lb ___ reps Set 2: ___ lb ___ reps Set 3: ___ lb ___ reps
BARBELL HACK SQUAT: 3 sets of 5–7 reps	Set 1: ___ lb ___ reps Set 2: ___ lb ___ reps Set 3: ___ lb ___ reps
STIFF-LEG DEADLIFT: 2 sets of 5–7 reps	Set 1: ___ lb ___ reps Set 2: ___ lb ___ reps
OVERHEAD DUMBBELL SQUAT: 2 sets of 5–7 reps	Set 1: ___ lb ___ reps Set 2: ___ lb ___ reps
LEG PRESS: 2 sets of 5–7 reps	Set 1: ___ lb ___ reps Set 2: ___ lb ___ reps
5-MINUTE CARDIOVASCULAR COOLDOWN:	Bicycling, walking, rowing, or stairclimbing

■ DAY 30: TUESDAY

MEAL 1: Denver Omelet (page 170), $\frac{1}{2}$ avocado, 1 or 2 fish-oil capsules, 1 cup green tea

MEAL 2: Any Metabolism Advantage Super Shake (page 172), 1 or 2 fish-oil capsules, $\frac{1}{2}$ teaspoon creatine

MEAL 3: Leftover Meta Meat Loaf from previous day, Mixed-Bean Salad (page 180), 1 or 2 fish-oil capsules

MEAL 4: Any Metabolism Advantage Super Shake (page 172), 1 or 2 fish-oil capsules, $\frac{1}{2}$ teaspoon creatine

MEAL 5 (DURING WORKOUT): $\frac{1}{2}$ recovery drink

MEAL 6 (POSTWORKOUT): $\frac{1}{2}$ recovery drink

MEAL 7: Salmon in Basil Cream Sauce (page 193), Toasted Quinoa Salad (page 176), 1 or 2 fish-oil capsules, 1 cup green tea

Interval Workout #1

5-MINUTE LOW-INTENSITY WARMUP

INTERVALS:
30 seconds at high intensity,
90 seconds at low intensity

Perform 10 total intervals

5-MINUTE LOW-INTENSITY COOLDOWN

DAY 31: WEDNESDAY

Meal Plan

MEAL 1: Spinach and Cheese Omelet (page 168), 1 orange, 1 or 2 fish-oil capsules, 1 cup green tea

MEAL 2: Any Metabolism Advantage Super Shake (page 172), 1 or 2 fish-oil capsules, ½ teaspoon creatine

MEAL 3: Chunks of leftover Basil Salmon from previous day, sprinkled on Metabolism Advantage Salad (page 175) with either Metabolism Advantage dressing (page 182), 1 or 2 fish-oil capsules

MEAL 4: Any Metabolism Advantage Super Shake (page 172), 1 or 2 fish-oil capsules, ½ teaspoon creatine

MEAL 5 (DURING WORKOUT): ½ recovery drink

MEAL 6 (POSTWORKOUT): ½ recovery drink

MEAL 7: 10 percent meal, 1 or 2 fish-oil capsules, 1 cup green tea

Upper-Body Strengthening Workout (page 122)

5-MINUTE CARDIOVASCULAR WARMUP:	Bicycling, walking, rowing, or stairclimbing
CHINUP: 4 sets of 5–7 reps (1 set with wide overhand grip, 1 set with narrow underhand grip, 1 set with left hand in overhand grip and right hand in underhand grip, 1 set with right hand in overhand grip and left hand in underhand grip)	Set 1 (wide overhand grip): ___ reps Set 2 (narrow underhand grip): ___ reps Set 3 (left hand in overhand grip and right hand in underhand grip): ___ reps Set 4 (right hand in overhand grip and left hand in underhand grip): ___ reps
ALTERNATING DUMBBELL INCLINE PRESS: 1 set with underhand grip, 2 sets with overhand grip	Set 1 (underhand grip): ___ lb ___ reps Set 2 (overhand grip): ___ lb ___ reps Set 3 (overhand grip): ___ lb ___ reps
BARBELL CLEAN: 2 sets of 5–7 reps	Set 1: ___ lb ___ reps Set 2: ___ lb ___ reps
ALTERNATING DUMBBELL SHOULDER PRESS ON SWISS BALL: 2 sets of 5–7 reps with each arm	Set 1 (right arm): ___ lb ___ reps Set 1 (left arm): ___ lb ___ reps Set 2 (right arm): ___ lb ___ reps Set 2 (left arm): ___ lb ___ reps

ALTERNATING DUMBBELL CURL ON SWISS BALL: 2 sets of 5–7 reps with each arm	Set 1 (right arm): ___ lb ___ reps Set 1 (left arm): ___ lb ___ reps Set 2 (right arm): ___ lb ___ reps Set 2 (left arm): ___ lb ___ reps
CLOSE-GRIP BENCH PRESS: 2 sets of 5–7 reps	Set 1: ___ lb ___ reps Set 2: ___ lb ___ reps
5-MINUTE CARDIOVASCULAR COOLDOWN:	Bicycling, walking, rowing, or stairclimbing

■ DAY 32: THURSDAY

WEEK 5

Meal Plan

MEAL 1: Asian Scrambled Eggs (page 168), 1 green apple, 1 or 2 fish-oil capsules, 1 cup green tea

MEAL 2: Any Metabolism Advantage Super Shake (page 172), 1 or 2 fish-oil capsules, $\frac{1}{2}$ teaspoon creatine

MEAL 3: Roasted chicken breast, Mediterranean Salad (page 176), 1 or 2 fish-oil capsules

MEAL 4: Any Metabolism Advantage Super Shake (page 172), 1 or 2 fish-oil capsules, $\frac{1}{2}$ teaspoon creatine

MEAL 5 (DURING WORKOUT): $\frac{1}{2}$ recovery drink

MEAL 6 (POSTWORKOUT): $\frac{1}{2}$ recovery drink

MEAL 7: Pecan-Crusted Salmon (page 194), Metabolism Advantage Salad (page 175) with either Metabolism Advantage dressing (page 182), 1 or 2 fish-oil capsules, 1 cup green tea

Interval Workout #2

5-MINUTE LOW-INTENSITY WARMUP	
INTERVALS: 60 seconds at high intensity, 60 seconds at low intensity	Perform 10 total intervals
5-MINUTE LOW-INTENSITY COOLDOWN	

■ DAY 33: FRIDAY

Meal Plan

MEAL 1: Greek Omelet (page 167), 1 orange, 1 or 2 fish-oil capsules, 1 cup green tea

MEAL 2: Any Metabolism Advantage Super Shake (page 172), 1 or 2 fish-oil capsules, $\frac{1}{2}$ teaspoon creatine

MEAL 3: Leftover Pecan-Crusted Salmon crumbled on leftover Metabolism Advantage Salad from previous day, 1 or 2 fish-oil capsules

MEAL 4: Any Metabolism Advantage Super Shake (page 172), 1 or 2 fish-oil capsules, $\frac{1}{2}$ teaspoon creatine

MEAL 5 (DURING WORKOUT): $\frac{1}{2}$ recovery drink

MEAL 6 (POSTWORKOUT): $\frac{1}{2}$ recovery drink

MEAL 7: Extra-Lean Beef Meatballs (page 200), Carrot Salad (page 178), Fruit Salad (page 178), 1 cup green tea

Total-Body Strengthening Workout (page 129)

5-MINUTE CARDIOVASCULAR WARMUP:	Bicycling, walking, rowing, or stairclimbing
SUITCASE DEADLIFT: 3 sets of 8–10 reps on each side	Set 1 (right side): ___ reps Set 1 (left side): ___ reps Set 2 (right side): ___ reps Set 2 (left side): ___ reps Set 3 (right side): ___ reps Set 3 (left side): ___ reps
DUMBBELL OVERHEAD WALKING LUNGE: 3 sets of 8–10 reps with each leg	Set 1: ___ lb ___ reps per leg Set 2: ___ lb ___ reps per leg Set 3: ___ lb ___ reps per leg
PUSH PRESS: 3 sets of 8–10 reps	Set 1: ___ lb ___ reps Set 2: ___ lb ___ reps Set 3: ___ lb ___ reps
BENT-OVER BARBELL ROW: 2 sets of 8–10 reps	Set 1: ___ lb ___ reps Set 2: ___ lb ___ reps
BRIDGE: 2 sets of 30 seconds each	Set 1: ___ Set 2: ___
SIDE BRIDGE: 2 sets on each side	Set 1 (right side): ___ Set 1 (left side): ___ Set 2 (right side): ___ Set 2 (left side): ___
5-MINUTE CARDIOVASCULAR COOLDOWN:	Bicycling, walking, rowing, or stairclimbing

DAY 34: SATURDAY (ASSUMING AM WORKOUT)

Meal Plan

MEAL 1 (DURING WORKOUT): $\frac{1}{2}$ recovery drink

MEAL 2 (POSTWORKOUT): $\frac{1}{2}$ recovery drink

MEAL 3: Mexican Frittata (page 170), $\frac{1}{2}$ avocado or Guacamole (page 180), 1 or 2 fish-oil capsules, 1 cup green tea

MEAL 4: Any Metabolism Advantage Super Shake (page 172), 1 or 2 fish-oil capsules, $\frac{1}{2}$ teaspoon creatine

MEAL 5: Quick Quinoa and Chicken (page 186), Mixed-Bean Salad (page 180), 1 or 2 fish-oil capsules

MEAL 6: 10 percent meal, 1 or 2 fish-oil capsules, 1 cup green tea

MEAL 7: Any Metabolism Advantage Super Shake (page 172), 1 or 2 fish-oil capsules, $\frac{1}{2}$ teaspoon creatine

Interval Workout #3

5-MINUTE LOW-INTENSITY WARMUP

INTERVALS: Perform 5 total intervals
90 seconds at high intensity,
180 seconds at low intensity

5-MINUTE LOW-INTENSITY COOLDOWN

DAY 35: SUNDAY (ASSUMING NO WORKOUT)

Meal Plan

MEAL 1: 10 percent meal, 1 or 2 fish-oil capsules, 1 cup green tea

MEAL 2: Extra-Lean Beef Meatballs (page 200), Metabolism Advantage Salad (page 175) with either Metabolism Advantage dressing (page 182), 1 or 2 fish-oil capsules, 1 cup green tea

MEAL 3: Any Metabolism Advantage Super Shake (page 172), 1 or 2 fish-oil capsules, $\frac{1}{2}$ teaspoon creatine

MEAL 4: Striped Bass with Artichoke and Asparagus (page 198), 1 or 2 fish-oil capsules, 1 cup green tea

MEAL 5: Snack or Bar (page 202), 1 cup green tea

Shopping List

DRY GOODS

- ❏ 3 cans (15½ ounces each) mixed beans (kidney beans, black beans, chickpeas), plus 3 cans (15½ ounces each) chickpeas
- ❏ 1 can (15½ ounces) sliced black olives, preferably Greek
- ❏ 1 can (8 ounces) juice-packed pineapple chunks
- ❏ 1 can (8 ounces) roasted red peppers
- ❏ 1 can (5 ounces) water chestnuts
- ❏ 1 can (14 ounces) artichoke hearts

PRODUCE

- ❏ 5 oranges
- ❏ 1 head iceberg lettuce
- ❏ 1 pound fresh spinach
- ❏ 4–5 ounces bean sprouts
- ❏ 8 ounces fresh mushrooms
- ❏ 2 or 3 heads garlic
- ❏ ½ head cabbage
- ❏ 4 carrots
- ❏ ½ pound baby carrots
- ❏ 2 large cucumbers
- ❏ 3 medium green bell peppers
- ❏ 1 red bell pepper
- ❏ 2 small jalapeños or 2 cans (4 ounces each) sliced jalapeños
- ❏ 2-inch piece fresh ginger
- ❏ 2 limes
- ❏ 5 large lemons
- ❏ 8 medium tomatoes
- ❏ 1 Roma tomato
- ❏ 1½ pounds broccoli
- ❏ 1 large head cauliflower
- ❏ 1 bunch celery
- ❏ 2 avocados (plus 3 more if you want homemade guacamole)
- ❏ 5 onions
- ❏ 1 red onion
- ❏ 11 medium scallions
- ❏ 5 snow peas
- ❏ 20 large asparagus spears, plus 1 pound
- ❏ 1 bunch fresh rosemary
- ❏ 1 bunch fresh cilantro
- ❏ 3 bunches fresh parsley
- ❏ 1 bunch fresh mint
- ❏ 4 ounces fresh or frozen green beans

REFRIGERATED ITEMS

- ❏ 3 large containers (32 ounces each) pasteurized egg whites
- ❏ 1 dozen omega-3 eggs
- ❏ 2 ounces feta cheese
- ❏ 8 ounces low-fat cottage cheese
- ❏ 1 container (8 ounces) low-fat, lactose-free plain yogurt

MEAT AND FISH

- ❏ 2½ pounds boneless, skinless chicken breasts
- ❏ 2 pounds extra-lean (96%) ground beef
- ❏ 4 ounces turkey ham
- ❏ 1 pound salmon fillets
- ❏ 1 can (14¾ ounces) salmon
- ❏ 1½ pounds striped bass fillets, with skin
- ❏ 6 ounces lean turkey sausage

CONDIMENTS, SPICES, MISCELLANEOUS

❏ Ingredients for Snack or Bar (page 202) of your choice
❏ Ingredients for 13 Super Shakes (page 172) of your choice
❏ 1 container (32 ounces; approximately 10 servings) recovery drink
❏ Ingredients for 2 servings of 10 percent meal

CHECK QUANTITIES AND FRESHNESS OF:

❏ Butter, coconut oil, or Smart Balance spread (need 6 tablespoons)
❏ Fish-oil capsules
❏ Green tea
❏ Quinoa (need 2½ cups)
❏ Oat bran (need ¾ cup)
❏ Wheat bran (need ⅛ cup)
❏ Flaxseed (need 2 tablespoons whole, ¼ cup ground, ¼ cup meal)
❏ Shelled mixed nuts (walnuts, almonds, pecans, cashews; need ⅔ cup mixed plus ½ cup walnuts)
❏ Shredded Colby cheese (need ½ cup)
❏ Shredded Cheddar cheese (need ¼ cup)
❏ Mozzarella cheese (need 1 slice)
❏ Fat-free American cheese (need 1 slice)
❏ Salsa (need ¼ cup)
❏ White cooking wine (need 2 tablespoons)
❏ Dry white wine (need 1½ tablespoons)

Goal Setting

Look back over your results from the previous week. If you got all your workouts in, give yourself a pat on the back. If not, list three ways you can increase your success in the coming week.

1. _____

_____

2. _____

_____

3. _____

_____

Week 6

■ **DAY 36: MONDAY**

Meal Plan

MEAL 1: The Big Omelet (page 171), 1 orange, 1 or 2 fish-oil capsules, 1 cup green tea

MEAL 2: Any Metabolism Advantage Super Shake (page 172), 1 or 2 fish-oil capsules, ½ teaspoon creatine

MEAL 3: Teriyaki Lettuce Wrap (page 184), roasted red peppers, 1 or 2 fish-oil capsules

MEAL 4: Any Metabolism Advantage Super Shake (page 172), 1 or 2 fish-oil capsules, ½ teaspoon creatine

MEAL 5 (DURING WORKOUT): ½ recovery drink

MEAL 6 (POSTWORKOUT): ½ recovery drink

MEAL 7: Thai Ground Beef (page 199), Metabolism Advantage Salad (page 175) with either Metabolism Advantage dressing (page 182), Toasted Quinoa Salad (page 176), 1 or 2 fish-oil capsules, 1 cup green tea

Lower-Body Strengthening Workout (page 117)

5-MINUTE CARDIOVASCULAR WARMUP:	Bicycling, walking, rowing, or stairclimbing
BARBELL GOOD MORNING: 3 sets of 5–7 reps	Set 1: ___ lb ___ reps Set 2: ___ lb ___ reps Set 3: ___ lb ___ reps
BARBELL HACK SQUAT: 3 sets of 5–7 reps	Set 1: ___ lb ___ reps Set 2: ___ lb ___ reps Set 3: ___ lb ___ reps
STIFF-LEG DEADLIFT: 2 sets of 5–7 reps	Set 1: ___ lb ___ reps Set 2: ___ lb ___ reps
OVERHEAD DUMBBELL SQUAT: 2 sets of 5–7 reps	Set 1: ___ lb ___ reps Set 2: ___ lb ___ reps
LEG PRESS: 2 sets of 5–7 reps	Set 1: ___ lb ___ reps Set 2: ___ lb ___ reps
5-MINUTE CARDIOVASCULAR COOLDOWN:	Bicycling, walking, rowing, or stairclimbing

DAY 37: TUESDAY

Meal Plan

MEAL 1: Greek Omelet (page 167), 1 orange, 1 or 2 fish-oil capsules, 1 cup green tea

MEAL 2: Any Metabolism Advantage Super Shake (page 172), 1 or 2 fish-oil capsules, ½ teaspoon creatine

MEAL 3: Roasted chicken breast, Hummus (page 179) with celery sticks, 1 or 2 fish-oil capsules

MEAL 4: Any Metabolism Advantage Super Shake (page 172), 1 or 2 fish-oil capsules, ½ teaspoon creatine

MEAL 5 (DURING WORKOUT): ½ recovery drink

MEAL 6 (POSTWORKOUT): ½ recovery drink

MEAL 7: Rosemary Salmon and Asparagus on the Grill (page 192), Mashed Garlic Cauliflower (page 181), 1 or 2 fish-oil capsules, 1 cup green tea

Interval Workout #1

5-MINUTE LOW-INTENSITY WARMUP

INTERVALS: Perform 10 total intervals
30 seconds at high intensity,
90 seconds at low intensity

5-MINUTE LOW-INTENSITY COOLDOWN

DAY 38: WEDNESDAY

Meal Plan

MEAL 1: Spinach and Cheese Omelet (page 168), 1 orange, 1 or 2 fish-oil capsules, 1 cup green tea

MEAL 2: Any Metabolism Advantage Super Shake (page 172), 1 or 2 fish-oil capsules, ½ teaspoon creatine

MEAL 3: Leftover Rosemary Salmon from previous day, crumbled on Metabolism Advantage Salad (page 175) with either Metabolism Advantage dressing (page 182), 1 or 2 fish-oil capsules

MEAL 4: Any Metabolism Advantage Super Shake (page 172), 1 or 2 fish-oil capsules, 1/2 teaspoon creatine

MEAL 5 (DURING WORKOUT): ½ recovery drink

MEAL 6 (POSTWORKOUT): ½ recovery drink

MEAL 7: Meta Meat Loaf (page 201), leftover Toasted Quinoa Salad from Monday, 1 or 2 fish-oil capsules, 1 cup green tea

Upper-Body Strengthening Workout (page 122)

5-MINUTE CARDIOVASCULAR WARMUP:	Bicycling, walking, rowing, or stairclimbing
CHINUP: 4 sets of 5–7 reps (1 set with wide overhand grip, 1 set with narrow underhand grip, 1 set with left hand in overhand grip and right hand in underhand grip, 1 set with right hand in overhand grip and left hand in underhand grip)	Set 1 (wide overhand grip): ___ reps Set 2 (narrow underhand grip): ___ reps Set 3 (left hand in overhand grip and right hand in underhand grip): ___ reps Set 4 (right hand in overhand grip and left hand in underhand grip): ___ reps
ALTERNATING DUMBBELL INCLINE PRESS: 1 set with underhand grip, 2 sets with overhand grip	Set 1 (underhand grip): ___ lb ___ reps Set 2 (overhand grip): ___ lb ___ reps Set 3 (overhand grip): ___ lb ___ reps
BARBELL CLEAN: 2 sets of 5–7 reps	Set 1: ___ lb ___ reps Set 2: ___ lb ___ reps
ALTERNATING DUMBBELL SHOULDER PRESS ON SWISS BALL: 2 sets of 5–7 reps with each arm	Set 1 (right arm): ___ lb ___ reps Set 1 (left arm): ___ lb ___ reps Set 2 (right arm): ___ lb ___ reps Set 2 (left arm): ___ lb ___ reps

ALTERNATING DUMBBELL CURL ON SWISS BALL: 2 sets of 5–7 reps with each arm	Set 1 (right arm): ___ lb ___ reps Set 1 (left arm): ___ lb ___ reps Set 2 (right arm): ___ lb ___ reps Set 2 (left arm): ___ lb ___ reps
CLOSE-GRIP BENCH PRESS: 2 sets of 5–7 reps	Set 1: ___ lb ___ reps Set 2: ___ lb ___ reps
5-MINUTE CARDIOVASCULAR COOLDOWN:	Bicycling, walking, rowing, or stairclimbing

■ DAY 39: THURSDAY

WEEK 6

Meal Plan

MEAL 1: Denver Omelet (page 170), 1 orange, 1 or 2 fish-oil capsules, 1 cup green tea

MEAL 2: Any Metabolism Advantage Super Shake (page 172), 1 or 2 fish-oil capsules, ½ teaspoon creatine

MEAL 3: Leftover Meta Meat Loaf from previous day, Mediterranean Salad (page 176), 1 or 2 fish-oil capsules

MEAL 4: Any Metabolism Advantage Super Shake (page 172), 1 or 2 fish-oil capsules, ½ teaspoon creatine

MEAL 5 (DURING WORKOUT): ½ recovery drink

MEAL 6 (POSTWORKOUT): ½ recovery drink

MEAL 7: Thai Ground Beef (page 199), Carrot Salad (page 178), 1 or 2 fish-oil capsules, 1 cup green tea

Interval Workout #2

5-MINUTE LOW-INTENSITY WARMUP	
INTERVALS: 60 seconds at high intensity, 60 seconds at low intensity	Perform 10 total intervals
5-MINUTE LOW-INTENSITY COOLDOWN	

■ DAY 40: FRIDAY

Meal Plan

MEAL 1: Asian Scrambled Eggs (page 168), 1 orange, 1 or 2 fish-oil capsules, 1 cup green tea

MEAL 2: Any Metabolism Advantage Super Shake (page 172), 1 or 2 fish-oil capsules, $\frac{1}{2}$ teaspoon creatine

MEAL 3: Roasted chicken breast, Metabolism Advantage Tabbouleh (page 181), 1 or 2 fish-oil capsules

MEAL 4: Any Metabolism Advantage Super Shake (page 172), 1 or 2 fish-oil capsules, $\frac{1}{2}$ teaspoon creatine

MEAL 5 (DURING WORKOUT): $\frac{1}{2}$ recovery drink

MEAL 6 (POSTWORKOUT): $\frac{1}{2}$ recovery drink

MEAL 7: Salmon Burger Stroganoff (page 191), 1 or 2 fish-oil capsules, 1 cup green tea

Total-Body Strengthening Workout (page 129)

5-MINUTE CARDIOVASCULAR WARMUP:	Bicycling, walking, rowing, or stairclimbing
SUITCASE DEADLIFT: 3 sets of 8–10 reps on each side	Set 1 (right side): ___ reps Set 1 (left side): ___ reps Set 2 (right side): ___ reps Set 2 (left side): ___ reps Set 3 (right side): ___ reps Set 3 (left side): ___ reps
DUMBBELL OVERHEAD WALKING LUNGE: 3 sets of 8–10 reps with each leg	Set 1: ___ lb ___ reps per leg Set 2: ___ lb ___ reps per leg Set 3: ___ lb ___ reps per leg
PUSH PRESS: 3 sets of 8–10 reps	Set 1: ___ lb ___ reps Set 2: ___ lb ___ reps Set 3: ___ lb ___ reps
BENT-OVER BARBELL ROW: 2 sets of 8–10 reps	Set 1: ___ lb ___ reps Set 2: ___ lb ___ reps
BRIDGE: 2 sets of 30 seconds each	Set 1: ___ Set 2: ___
SIDE BRIDGE: 2 sets on each side	Set 1 (right side): ___ Set 1 (left side): ___ Set 2 (right side): ___ Set 2 (left side): ___
5-MINUTE CARDIOVASCULAR COOLDOWN:	Bicycling, walking, rowing, or stairclimbing

■ DAY 41: SATURDAY (ASSUMING AM WORKOUT)

Meal Plan

MEAL 1 (DURING WORKOUT): $\frac{1}{2}$ recovery drink

MEAL 2 (POSTWORKOUT): $\frac{1}{2}$ recovery drink

MEAL 3: Mexican Frittata (page 170), $\frac{1}{2}$ avocado or Guacamole (page 180), 1 or 2 fish-oil capsules, 1 cup green tea

MEAL 4: Any Metabolism Advantage Super Shake (page 172), 1 or 2 fish-oil capsules, $\frac{1}{2}$ teaspoon creatine

MEAL 5: Quick Quinoa and Chicken (page 186), Mixed-Bean Salad (page 180), 1 or 2 fish-oil capsules

MEAL 6: 10 percent meal, 1 or 2 fish-oil capsules, 1 cup green tea

MEAL 7: Any Metabolism Advantage Super Shake (page 172), 1 or 2 fish-oil capsules, $\frac{1}{2}$ teaspoon creatine

Interval Workout #3

5-MINUTE LOW-INTENSITY WARMUP

INTERVALS:	Perform 5 total intervals
90 seconds at high intensity, 180 seconds at low intensity	

5-MINUTE LOW-INTENSITY COOLDOWN

■ DAY 42: SUNDAY (ASSUMING NO WORKOUT)

Meal Plan

MEAL 1: 10 percent meal, 1 or 2 fish-oil capsules, 1 cup green tea

MEAL 2: Extra-Lean Beef Meatballs (page 200), Metabolism Advantage Salad (page 175) with either Metabolism Advantage dressing (page 182), 1 or 2 fish-oil capsules, 1 cup green tea

MEAL 3: Any Metabolism Advantage Super Shake (page 172), 1 or 2 fish-oil capsules, $\frac{1}{2}$ teaspoon creatine

MEAL 4: Striped Bass with Artichoke and Asparagus (page 198), 1 or 2 fish-oil capsules, 1 cup green tea

MEAL 5: Snack or Bar (page 202), 1 cup green tea

Shopping List

DRY GOODS

❏ 6 cans (15½ ounces each) mixed beans (kidney beans, black beans, chickpeas), plus 3 cans (15½ ounces each) chickpeas

❏ 1 can (15½ ounces) sliced black olives, preferably Greek

❏ 1 can (5 ounces) juice-packed pineapple chunks

❏ 1 can (14 ounces) artichoke hearts (or 1 package frozen)

PRODUCE

❏ 3 oranges
❏ 1 green apple
❏ ¼ pint strawberries
❏ 1 medium banana
❏ 1 large kiwifruit
❏ 1 bunch fresh cilantro
❏ 2 pounds fresh spinach
❏ 4 ounces fresh mushrooms
❏ 1 red bell pepper
❏ 1 green bell pepper
❏ 1 Roma tomato
❏ 10 tomatoes
❏ 3 pounds broccoli
❏ 1 bunch celery
❏ 1 large head cauliflower
❏ 1 pound asparagus
❏ 4 avocados (plus 3 more if you want homemade guacamole)

❏ 1 pound baby carrots
❏ 4–6 large carrots
❏ 4 ounces fresh or frozen green beans
❏ 1 bunch fresh mint
❏ 1 bunch fresh cilantro
❏ 1 bunch fresh basil
❏ 1 bunch fresh parsley
❏ 2 or 3 shallots
❏ 1 red onion
❏ 1 small jalapeño or 1 can (4 ounces) sliced jalapeños
❏ 1-inch piece fresh ginger
❏ 1 lime
❏ 3 lemons
❏ 2 heads garlic
❏ 4 onions

REFRIGERATED ITEMS

❏ 3 large containers (32 ounces each) pasteurized egg whites
❏ ½ dozen omega-3 eggs
❏ 4 ounces feta cheese

❏ 1 cup shredded Colby cheese
❏ 4 ounces Parmesan cheese
❏ 2 containers (8 ounces each) low-fat, lactose-free plain yogurt

MEATS AND FISH

❏ 1 pound, 10 ounces salmon fillets
❏ 1½ pounds striped bass fillets, with skin

❏ 1½ pounds sea scallops
❏ 8 ounces turkey sausage or 2 ounces turkey bacon

❑ 8 ounces turkey ham

❑ 1⅓ pound extra-lean (96%) ground beef

❑ 3½ pounds boneless, skinless chicken breasts

CONDIMENTS, SPICES, MISCELLANEOUS

❑ Ingredients for 11 Super Shakes (page 172) of your choice

❑ Ingredients for Snack or Bar (page 202) of your choice

❑ 1 container (32 ounces; approximately 10 servings) recovery drink

❑ Ingredients for 2 servings of 10 percent meal

CHECK QUANTITIES AND FRESHNESS OF:

❑ Shelled mixed nuts (walnuts, almonds, pecans, cashews); need 1⅛ cups mixed, ½ cup almonds, ¼ cup walnuts, 2 tablespoons pecan meal

❑ Quinoa (need 1½ cups)

❑ Flaxseed (need ⅛ cup ground)

❑ Fish-oil capsules

❑ Green tea

❑ Wheat bran (need ⅛ cup)

❑ Shredded Cheddar cheese (need ¼ cup)

❑ Fat-free American cheese (need 2 slices)

❑ Mozzarella cheese (need 1 slice)

❑ Raisins (need ½ cup)

❑ Cooking wine (need ⅓ cup)

❑ Dry white wine (need 1½ tablespoons)

❑ Salsa (need ¼ cup)

❑ Butter, coconut oil, or Smart Balance spread

Goal Setting

Look back over your results from the previous week. If you got all your workouts in, give yourself a pat on the back. If not, list three ways you can increase your success in the coming week.

1. _____

_____

2. _____

_____

3. _____

_____

Week 7

DAY 43: MONDAY

Meal Plan

MEAL 1: Greek Omelet (page 167), 1 orange, 1 or 2 fish-oil capsules, 1 cup green tea

MEAL 2: Any Metabolism Advantage Super Shake (page 172), 1 or 2 fish-oil capsules, ½ teaspoon creatine

MEAL 3: Leftover Striped Bass from previous day, crumbled on Metabolism Advantage Salad (page 175) with either Metabolism Advantage dressing (page 182), 1 or 2 fish-oil capsules

MEAL 4: Any Metabolism Advantage Super Shake (page 172), 1 or 2 fish-oil capsules, ½ teaspoon creatine

MEAL 5 (DURING WORKOUT): ½ recovery drink

MEAL 6 (POSTWORKOUT): ½ recovery drink

MEAL 7: Pecan-Crusted Salmon (page 194), Mashed Garlic Cauliflower (page 181), Toasted Quinoa Salad (page 176), Fruit Salad (page 178), 1 or 2 fish-oil capsules, 1 cup green tea

Lower-Body Strengthening Workout (page 117)

5-MINUTE CARDIOVASCULAR WARMUP:	Bicycling, walking, rowing, or stairclimbing
BARBELL GOOD MORNING: 3 sets of 5–7 reps	Set 1: ___ lb ___ reps Set 2: ___ lb ___ reps Set 3: ___ lb ___ reps
BARBELL HACK SQUAT: 3 sets of 5–7 reps	Set 1: ___ lb ___ reps Set 2: ___ lb ___ reps Set 3: ___ lb ___ reps
STIFF-LEG DEADLIFT: 2 sets of 5–7 reps	Set 1: ___ lb ___ reps Set 2: ___ lb ___ reps
OVERHEAD DUMBBELL SQUAT: 2 sets of 5–7 reps	Set 1: ___ lb ___ reps Set 2: ___ lb ___ reps
LEG PRESS: 2 sets of 5–7 reps	Set 1: ___ lb ___ reps Set 2: ___ lb ___ reps
5-MINUTE CARDIOVASCULAR COOLDOWN:	Bicycling, walking, rowing, or stairclimbing

DAY 44: TUESDAY

Meal Plan

MEAL 1: Denver Omelet (page 170), ½ avocado, 1 or 2 fish-oil capsules, 1 cup green tea

MEAL 2: Any Metabolism Advantage Super Shake (page 172), 1 or 2 fish-oil capsules, ½ teaspoon creatine

MEAL 3: Leftover Pecan-Crusted Salmon crumbled on leftover Metabolism Advantage Salad from previous day, 1 or 2 fish-oil capsules

MEAL 4: Any Metabolism Advantage Super Shake (page 172), 1 or 2 fish-oil capsules, ½ teaspoon creatine

MEAL 5 (DURING WORKOUT): ½ recovery drink

MEAL 6 (POSTWORKOUT): ½ recovery drink

MEAL 7: Roasted Chicken with Rosemary Wheat Berries (page 186), leftover Toasted Quinoa Salad, 1 or 2 fish-oil capsules, 1 cup green tea

Interval Workout #1

5-MINUTE LOW-INTENSITY WARMUP

INTERVALS:
30 seconds at high intensity,
90 seconds at low intensity

Perform 10 total intervals

5-MINUTE LOW-INTENSITY COOLDOWN

DAY 45: WEDNESDAY

Meal Plan

MEAL 1: The Big Omelet (page 171), 1 orange, 1 or 2 fish-oil capsules, 1 cup green tea

MEAL 2: Any Metabolism Advantage Super Shake (page 172), 1 or 2 fish-oil capsules, ½ teaspoon creatine

MEAL 3: Roasted chicken breast, Hummus (page 179) with celery sticks, 1 or 2 fish-oil capsules

MEAL 4: Any Metabolism Advantage Super Shake (page 172), 1 or 2 fish-oil capsules, ½ teaspoon creatine

MEAL 5 (DURING WORKOUT): ½ recovery drink

MEAL 6 (POSTWORKOUT): ½ recovery drink

MEAL 7: Salmon in Basil Cream Sauce (page 193), Metabolism Advantage Salad (page 175) with either Metabolism Advantage dressing (page 182), Carrot Salad (page 178), 1 or 2 fish-oil capsules, 1 cup green tea

Upper-Body Strengthening Workout (page 122)

5-MINUTE CARDIOVASCULAR WARMUP:	Bicycling, walking, rowing, or stairclimbing
CHINUP: 4 sets of 5–7 reps (1 set with wide overhand grip, 1 set with narrow underhand grip, 1 set with left hand in overhand grip and right hand in underhand grip, 1 set with right hand in overhand grip and left hand in underhand grip)	Set 1 (wide overhand grip): ___ reps Set 2 (narrow underhand grip): ___ reps Set 3 (left hand in overhand grip and right hand in underhand grip): ___ reps Set 4 (right hand in overhand grip and left hand in underhand grip): ___ reps
ALTERNATING DUMBBELL INCLINE PRESS: 1 set with underhand grip, 2 sets with overhand grip	Set 1 (underhand grip): ___ lb ___ reps Set 2 (overhand grip): ___ lb ___ reps Set 3 (overhand grip): ___ lb ___ reps
BARBELL CLEAN: 2 sets of 5–7 reps	Set 1: ___ lb ___ reps Set 2: ___ lb ___ reps
ALTERNATING DUMBBELL SHOULDER PRESS ON SWISS BALL: 2 sets of 5–7 reps with each arm	Set 1 (right arm): ___ lb ___ reps Set 1 (left arm): ___ lb ___ reps Set 2 (right arm): ___ lb ___ reps Set 2 (left arm): ___ lb ___ reps

ALTERNATING DUMBBELL CURL ON SWISS BALL: 2 sets of 5–7 reps with each arm	Set 1 (right arm): ___ lb ___ reps Set 1 (left arm): ___ lb ___ reps Set 2 (right arm): ___ lb ___ reps Set 2 (left arm): ___ lb ___ reps
CLOSE-GRIP BENCH PRESS: 2 sets of 5–7 reps	Set 1: ___ lb ___ reps Set 2: ___ lb ___ reps
5-MINUTE CARDIOVASCULAR COOLDOWN:	Bicycling, walking, rowing, or stairclimbing

■ DAY 46: THURSDAY

Meal Plan

MEAL 1: Scrambled Eggs and Greens (page 169), 1 green apple, 1 or 2 fish-oil capsules, 1 cup green tea

MEAL 2: Any Metabolism Advantage Super Shake (page 172), 1 or 2 fish-oil capsules, ½ teaspoon creatine

MEAL 3: Leftover Basil Salmon crumbled on leftover Metabolism Advantage Salad from previous day, 1 or 2 fish-oil capsules

MEAL 4: Any Metabolism Advantage Super Shake (page 172), 1 or 2 fish-oil capsules, ½ teaspoon creatine

MEAL 5 (DURING WORKOUT): ½ recovery drink

MEAL 6 (POSTWORKOUT): ½ recovery drink

MEAL 7: Almond-Crusted Sea Scallops with Tomato-Onion Gratin (page 196), Toasted Quinoa Salad (page 176), 1 or 2 fish-oil capsules, 1 cup green tea

Interval Workout #2

5-MINUTE LOW-INTENSITY WARMUP	
INTERVALS: 60 seconds at high intensity, 60 seconds at low intensity	Perform 10 total intervals
5-MINUTE LOW-INTENSITY COOLDOWN	

■ DAY 47: FRIDAY

Meal Plan

MEAL 1: Spinach and Cheese Omelet (page 168), 1 orange, 1 or 2 fish-oil capsules, 1 cup green tea

MEAL 2: Any Metabolism Advantage Super Shake (page 172), 1 or 2 fish-oil capsules, ½ teaspoon creatine

MEAL 3: Roasted chicken, Metabolism Advantage Salad (page 175) with either Metabolism Advantage dressing (page 182), 1 or 2 fish-oil capsules

MEAL 4: Any Metabolism Advantage Super Shake (page 172), 1 or 2 fish-oil capsules, ½ teaspoon creatine

MEAL 5 (DURING WORKOUT): ½ recovery drink

MEAL 6 (POSTWORKOUT): ½ recovery drink

MEAL 7: Greek Burger (page 194), Carrot Salad (page 178), 1 or 2 fish-oil capsules, 1 cup green tea

Total-Body Strengthening Workout (page 129)

5-MINUTE CARDIOVASCULAR WARMUP:	Bicycling, walking, rowing, or stairclimbing
SUITCASE DEADLIFT: 3 sets of 8–10 reps on each side	Set 1 (right side): ___ reps Set 1 (left side): ___ reps Set 2 (right side): ___ reps Set 2 (left side): ___ reps Set 3 (right side): ___ reps Set 3 (left side): ___ reps
DUMBBELL OVERHEAD WALKING LUNGE: 3 sets of 8–10 reps with each leg	Set 1: ___ lb ___ reps per leg Set 2: ___ lb ___ reps per leg Set 3: ___ lb ___ reps per leg
PUSH PRESS: 3 sets of 8–10 reps	Set 1: ___ lb ___ reps Set 2: ___ lb ___ reps Set 3: ___ lb ___ reps
BENT-OVER BARBELL ROW: 2 sets of 8–10 reps	Set 1: ___ lb ___ reps Set 2: ___ lb ___ reps
BRIDGE: 2 sets of 30 seconds each	Set 1: ___ Set 2: ___
SIDE BRIDGE: 2 sets on each side	Set 1 (right side): ___ Set 1 (left side): ___ Set 2 (right side): ___ Set 2 (left side): ___
5-MINUTE CARDIOVASCULAR COOLDOWN:	Bicycling, walking, rowing, or stairclimbing

■ DAY 48: SATURDAY (ASSUMING AM WORKOUT)

Meal Plan

MEAL 1 (DURING WORKOUT): ½ recovery drink

MEAL 2 (POSTWORKOUT): ½ recovery drink

MEAL 3: Mexican Frittata (page 170), ½ avocado or Guacamole (page 180), 1 or 2 fish-oil capsules, 1 cup green tea

MEAL 4: Any Metabolism Advantage Super Shake (page 172), 1 or 2 fish-oil capsules, 1/2 teaspoon creatine

MEAL 5: Quick Quinoa and Chicken (page 186), Mixed-Bean Salad (page 180), 1 or 2 fish-oil capsules

MEAL 6: 10 percent meal, 1 or 2 fish-oil capsules, 1 cup green tea

MEAL 7: Any Metabolism Advantage Super Shake (page 172), 1 or 2 fish-oil capsules, ½ teaspoon creatine

Interval Workout #3

5-MINUTE LOW-INTENSITY WARMUP

INTERVALS:	Perform 5 total intervals
90 seconds at high intensity, 180 seconds at low intensity	

5-MINUTE LOW-INTENSITY COOLDOWN

■ DAY 49: SUNDAY (ASSUMING NO WORKOUT)

Meal Plan

MEAL 1: 10 percent meal, 1 or 2 fish-oil capsules, 1 cup green tea

MEAL 2: Extra-Lean Beef Meatballs (page 200), Metabolism Advantage Salad (page 175) with either Metabolism Advantage dressing (page 182), 1 or 2 fish-oil capsules, 1 cup green tea

MEAL 3: Any Metabolism Advantage Super Shake (page 172), 1 or 2 fish-oil capsules, ½ teaspoon creatine

MEAL 4: Striped Bass with Artichoke and Asparagus (page 198), 1 or 2 fish-oil capsules, 1 cup green tea

MEAL 5: Snack or Bar (page 202), 1 cup green tea

SHOPPING LIST

DRY GOODS

❏ 3 cans (15½ ounces each) mixed beans (kidney beans, black beans, chickpeas), plus 1 can (15½ ounces) kidney beans

❏ 1 can (15½ ounces) sliced black olives, preferably Greek

❏ 1 can (5 ounces) water chestnuts

❏ 2 cans (8 ounces each) roasted red peppers

❏ 1 can (14 ounces) artichoke hearts (or 1 package frozen)

PRODUCE

❏ 4 oranges

❏ 12 ounces fresh mushrooms

❏ 1 large cucumber

❏ 1 large head cauliflower

❏ 1 head iceberg lettuce

❏ 20 large asparagus spears

❏ 1¼ pounds fresh spinach

❏ 7 tomatoes

❏ 1 Roma tomato

❏ 4–5 ounces bean sprouts

❏ 3 medium scallions

❏ ½ pound baby carrots

❏ 1 large carrot

❏ 3 avocados (plus 3 more if you want homemade guacamole)

❏ 1½ pounds broccoli

❏ 5 snow peas

❏ 3 bell peppers (any color), plus 1 yellow and 1 red

❏ 1 bunch fresh mint

❏ 1 red onion

❏ 2 small jalapeños or 2 cans (4 ounces each) sliced jalapeños

❏ 2-inch piece fresh ginger

❏ ¼ head cabbage

❏ 4 ounces fresh or frozen green beans

❏ 1 bunch fresh parsley

❏ 1 bunch fresh rosemary

❏ 1 pound asparagus

❏ 1 bunch fresh cilantro

❏ 2 large lemons

❏ Lime juice

❏ 2 heads garlic

❏ 4 onions

REFRIGERATED

❏ 3 large containers (32 ounces each) pasteurized egg whites

❏ 1 dozen omega-3 eggs

❏ 4 ounces feta cheese

❏ 1 container (8 ounces) low-fat, lactose-free plain yogurt

MEAT AND FISH

❏ 1½ pounds striped bass fillets, with skin

❏ 1 pound salmon fillets

❏ 1 can (14¾ ounces) salmon

❏ 3 pounds extra-lean (96%) ground beef

❏ 4½ pounds boneless, skinless chicken breasts

❏ 6 ounces lean turkey sausage

❏ 4 ounces turkey ham

CONDIMENTS, SPICES, MISCELLANEOUS

❑ Ingredients for 13 Super Shakes
(page 172) of your choice
❑ Ingredients for 1 Snack or Bar
(page 202) of your choice

❑ 1 container (32 ounces; approximately 10 servings) recovery drink
❑ Ingredients for 2 servings of
10 percent meal
❑ 2 packets chili powder

CHECK QUANTITIES AND FRESHNESS OF:

❑ Fish-oil capsules
❑ Green tea
❑ Quinoa (need 2½ cups)
❑ Flaxseed (need ⅛ cup ground and
¼ cup meal)
❑ Wheat bran (need ⅛ cup)
❑ Oat bran (need ¼ cup)
❑ Shelled mixed nuts (walnuts,
almonds, pecans, cashews; need
⅔ cup mixed, ½ cup walnuts, and
½ cup cashews)
❑ Shredded Colby cheese (need
½ cup)

❑ Shredded Cheddar cheese (need
¼ cup)
❑ Fat-free American cheese (need
2 slices)
❑ Spicy hot V8 (need 1 cup)
❑ Butter, coconut oil, or Smart
Balance spread
❑ Salsa (need ¼ cup)
❑ White cooking wine (need
2 tablespoons)
❑ Dry white wine (need
1½ tablespoons)

Goal Setting

Look back over your results from the previous week. If you got all your workouts in, give yourself a pat on the back. If not, list three ways you can increase your success in the coming week.

1. _____

_____

2. _____

_____

3. _____

_____

Week 8

◼ DAY 50: MONDAY

Meal Plan

MEAL 1: Asian Scrambled Eggs (page 168), 1 orange, 1 or 2 fish-oil capsules, 1 cup green tea

MEAL 2: Any Metabolism Advantage Super Shake (page 172), 1 or 2 fish-oil capsules, ½ teaspoon creatine

MEAL 3: Roasted chicken breast, roasted red peppers, 1 or 2 fish-oil capsules

MEAL 4: Any Metabolism Advantage Super Shake (page 172), 1 or 2 fish-oil capsules, ½ teaspoon creatine

MEAL 5 (DURING WORKOUT): ½ recovery drink

MEAL 6 (POSTWORKOUT): ½ recovery drink

MEAL 7: Rosemary Salmon and Asparagus on the Grill (page 192), Grilled Peppers and Tomatoes (page 177), Toasted Quinoa Salad (page 176), 1 or 2 fish-oil capsules, 1 cup green tea

Lower-Body Strengthening Workout (page 117)

5-MINUTE CARDIOVASCULAR WARMUP:	Bicycling, walking, rowing, or stairclimbing
BARBELL GOOD MORNING: 3 sets of 5–7 reps	Set 1: ___ lb ___ reps Set 2: ___ lb ___ reps Set 3: ___ lb ___ reps
BARBELL HACK SQUAT: 3 sets of 5–7 reps	Set 1: ___ lb ___ reps Set 2: ___ lb ___ reps Set 3: ___ lb ___ reps
STIFF-LEG DEADLIFT: 2 sets of 5–7 reps	Set 1: ___ lb ___ reps Set 2: ___ lb ___ reps
OVERHEAD DUMBBELL SQUAT: 2 sets of 5–7 reps	Set 1: ___ lb ___ reps Set 2: ___ lb ___ reps
LEG PRESS: 2 sets of 5–7 reps	Set 1: ___ lb ___ reps Set 2: ___ lb ___ reps
5-MINUTE CARDIOVASCULAR COOLDOWN:	Bicycling, walking, rowing, or stairclimbing

DAY 51: TUESDAY

Meal Plan

MEAL 1: The Big Omelet (page 171), 1 orange, 1 or 2 fish-oil capsules, 1 cup green tea

MEAL 2: Any Metabolism Advantage Super Shake (page 172), 1 or 2 fish-oil capsules, ½ teaspoon creatine

MEAL 3: Leftover rosemary salmon from previous day, crumbled onto Metabolism Advantage Salad (page 175) with either Metabolism Advantage dressing (page 182), 1 or 2 fish-oil capsules

MEAL 4: Any Metabolism Advantage Super Shake (page 172), 1 or 2 fish-oil capsules, ½ teaspoon creatine

MEAL 5 (DURING WORKOUT): ½ recovery drink

MEAL 6 (POSTWORKOUT): ½ recovery drink

MEAL 7: Thai Ground Beef (page 199), Toasted Quinoa Salad (page 176), 1 or 2 fish-oil capsules, 1 cup green tea

Interval Workout #1

5-MINUTE LOW-INTENSITY WARMUP

INTERVALS: Perform 10 total intervals
30 seconds at high intensity,
90 seconds at low intensity

5-MINUTE LOW-INTENSITY COOLDOWN

DAY 52: WEDNESDAY

MEAL 1: Denver Omelet (page 170), 1 orange, 1 or 2 fish-oil capsules, 1 cup green tea

MEAL 2: Any Metabolism Advantage Super Shake (page 172), 1 or 2 fish-oil capsules, ½ teaspoon creatine

MEAL 3: Roasted chicken breast, leftover Metabolism Advantage Salad from previous day, 1 or 2 fish-oil capsules

MEAL 4: Any Metabolism Advantage Super Shake (page 172), 1 or 2 fish-oil capsules, ½ teaspoon creatine

MEAL 5 (DURING WORKOUT): ½ recovery drink

MEAL 6 (POSTWORKOUT): ½ recovery drink

MEAL 7: Salmon Burger Stroganoff (page 191), leftover Toasted Quinoa Salad, 1 or 2 fish-oil capsules, 1 cup green tea

Upper-Body Strengthening Workout (page 122)

5-MINUTE CARDIOVASCULAR WARMUP:	Bicycling, walking, rowing, or stairclimbing
CHINUP: 4 sets of 5–7 reps (1 set with wide overhand grip, 1 set with narrow underhand grip, 1 set with left hand in overhand grip and right hand in underhand grip, 1 set with right hand in overhand grip and left hand in underhand grip)	Set 1 (wide overhand grip): ___ reps Set 2 (narrow underhand grip): ___ reps Set 3 (left hand in overhand grip and right hand in underhand grip): ___ reps Set 4 (right hand in overhand grip and left hand in underhand grip): ___ reps
ALTERNATING DUMBBELL INCLINE PRESS: 1 set with underhand grip, 2 sets with overhand grip	Set 1 (underhand grip): ___ lb ___ reps Set 2 (overhand grip): ___ lb ___ reps Set 3 (overhand grip): ___ lb ___ reps
BARBELL CLEAN: 2 sets of 5–7 reps	Set 1: ___ lb ___ reps Set 2: ___ lb ___ reps
ALTERNATING DUMBBELL SHOULDER PRESS ON SWISS BALL: 2 sets of 5–7 reps with each arm	Set 1 (right arm): ___ lb ___ reps Set 1 (left arm): ___ lb ___ reps Set 2 (right arm): ___ lb ___ reps Set 2 (left arm): ___ lb ___ reps

ALTERNATING DUMBBELL CURL ON SWISS BALL: 2 sets of 5–7 reps with each arm	Set 1 (right arm): ___ lb ___ reps Set 1 (left arm): ___ lb ___ reps Set 2 (right arm): ___ lb ___ reps Set 2 (left arm): ___ lb ___ reps
CLOSE-GRIP BENCH PRESS: 2 sets of 5–7 reps	Set 1: ___ lb ___ reps Set 2: ___ lb ___ reps
5-MINUTE CARDIOVASCULAR COOLDOWN:	Bicycling, walking, rowing, or stairclimbing

■ DAY 53: THURSDAY

Meal Plan

MEAL 1: Scrambled Eggs and Greens (page 169), ½ avocado, 1 or 2 fish-oil capsules, 1 cup green tea

MEAL 2: Any Metabolism Advantage Super Shake (page 172), 1 or 2 fish-oil capsules, ½ teaspoon creatine

MEAL 3: Roasted chicken breast (page 186), Mediterranean Salad (page 176), 1 or 2 fish-oil capsules

MEAL 4: Any Metabolism Advantage Super Shake (page 172), 1 or 2 fish-oil capsules, ½ teaspoon creatine

MEAL 5 (DURING WORKOUT): ½ recovery drink

MEAL 6 (POSTWORKOUT): ½ recovery drink

MEAL 7: Greek Burger (page 194), Mashed Garlic Cauliflower (page 181), 1 or 2 fish-oil capsules, 1 cup green tea

Interval Workout #2

5-MINUTE LOW-INTENSITY WARMUP	
INTERVALS: 60 seconds at high intensity, 60 seconds at low intensity	Perform 10 total intervals
5-MINUTE LOW-INTENSITY COOLDOWN	

DAY 54: FRIDAY

MEAL 1: Greek Omelet (page 167), 1 orange, 1 or 2 fish-oil capsules, 1 cup green tea

MEAL 2: Any Metabolism Advantage Super Shake (page 172), 1 or 2 fish-oil capsules, ½ teaspoon creatine

MEAL 3: Teriyaki Lettuce Wrap (page 184), roasted red peppers, 1 or 2 fish-oil capsules

MEAL 4: Any Metabolism Advantage Super Shake (page 172), 1 or 2 fish-oil capsules, ½ teaspoon creatine

MEAL 5 (DURING WORKOUT): ½ recovery drink

MEAL 6 (POSTWORKOUT): ½ recovery drink

MEAL 7: Chili in a Flash (page 200), leftover Toasted Quinoa Salad, 1 or 2 fish-oil capsules, 1 cup green tea

Total-Body Strengthening Workout (page 129)

5-MINUTE CARDIOVASCULAR WARMUP:	Bicycling, walking, rowing, or stairclimbing
SUITCASE DEADLIFT: 3 sets of 8–10 reps on each side	Set 1 (right side): ___ reps Set 1 (left side): ___ reps Set 2 (right side): ___ reps Set 2 (left side): ___ reps Set 3 (right side): ___ reps Set 3 (left side): ___ reps
DUMBBELL OVERHEAD WALKING LUNGE: 3 sets of 8–10 reps with each leg	Set 1: ___ lb ___ reps per leg Set 2: ___ lb ___ reps per leg Set 3: ___ lb ___ reps per leg
PUSH PRESS: 3 sets of 8–10 reps	Set 1: ___ lb ___ reps Set 2: ___ lb ___ reps Set 3: ___ lb ___ reps
BENT-OVER BARBELL ROW: 2 sets of 8–10 reps	Set 1: ___ lb ___ reps Set 2: ___ lb ___ reps
BRIDGE: 2 sets of 30 seconds each	Set 1: ___ Set 2: ___
SIDE BRIDGE: 2 sets on each side	Set 1 (right side): ___ Set 1 (left side): ___ Set 2 (right side): ___ Set 2 (left side): ___
5-MINUTE CARDIOVASCULAR COOLDOWN:	Bicycling, walking, rowing, or stairclimbing

DAY 55: SATURDAY (ASSUMING AM WORKOUT)

Meal Plan

MEAL 1 (DURING WORKOUT): ½ recovery drink

MEAL 2 (POSTWORKOUT): ½ recovery drink

MEAL 3: Mexican Frittata (page 170), ½ avocado or Guacamole (page 180), 1 or 2 fish-oil capsules, 1 cup green tea

MEAL 4: Any Metabolism Advantage Super Shake (page 172), 1 or 2 fish-oil capsules, ½ teaspoon creatine

MEAL 5: Quick Quinoa and Chicken (page 186), Mixed Bean Salad (page 180), 1 or 2 fish-oil capsules

MEAL 6: 10 percent meal, 1 or 2 fish-oil capsules, 1 cup green tea

MEAL 7: Any Metabolism Advantage Super Shake (page 172), 1 or 2 fish-oil capsules, ½ teaspoon creatine

Interval Workout #3

5-MINUTE LOW-INTENSITY WARMUP

INTERVALS:	Perform 5 total intervals
90 seconds at high intensity, 180 seconds at low intensity	

5-MINUTE LOW-INTENSITY COOLDOWN

DAY 56: SUNDAY (ASSUMING NO WORKOUT)

Meal Plan

MEAL 1: 10 percent meal, 1 or 2 fish-oil capsules, 1 cup green tea

MEAL 2: Extra-Lean Beef Meatballs (page 200), Metabolism Advantage Salad (page 175) with either Metabolism Advantage dressing (page 182), 1 or 2 fish-oil capsules, 1 cup green tea

MEAL 3: Any Metabolism Advantage Super Shake (page 172), 1 or 2 fish-oil capsules, ½ teaspoon creatine

MEAL 4: Striped Bass with Artichoke and Asparagus (page 198), 1 or 2 fish-oil capsules, 1 cup green tea

MEAL 5: Snack or Bar (page 202), 1 cup green tea

9

The Cheater's Guide

How to tweak the plan to match your lifestyle and interests

Many popular exercise and nutrition programs create the impression that there's only one way to burn fat, build muscle, and boost metabolism. Sure, they don't say it outright, but with their rigid programming, it's hard to believe that they're suggesting anything else. Take a look at reality (and research), however, and you'll see a very different picture. In practice, most people achieve better results when they customize a program to fit their lifestyles and goals.

In Chapter 8, you found one plan to help you get the Metabolism Advantage. That plan includes six exercise sessions a week, schedules your nutrient intake based on evening workouts, and assumes you can prepare most of your meals on your own. What if you can work out only 5 days a week? What if you'd prefer to spend more time in the weight room and less time on the treadmill, or vice versa? What if you routinely must eat out for business? What if you're using your oven for extra storage space? Does that mean you can't rev up your metabolism?

Not in the least!

The menus and exercise routines in Chapter 8 represent just one way to get the Metabolism Advantage, but it's certainly not the only way. When writing this book, I was presented with a challenge. I wanted to create one easy-to-follow program that anyone could use with success. Enter the day-by-day, very specific program in Chapter 8. At the same time, I also wanted to give you the tools to modify that program to fit the reality that is your life. That's what this chapter is all about.

In this chapter, you will learn how to:

1. Modify the strength and cardio workouts to fit your personal interests. In Chapter 5, you found a program that suggested three weight training and three cardio workouts a week. What if you'd rather spend an extra day running and one less day in the gym? No problem. What if you'd rather spend more time in the weight room and less time doing cardio? No problem there either. In this chapter, you'll find alternate workouts to help you do just that.
2. Eat out without going off the plan.

Changing Your Workouts to Fit Your Goals

Ever seen someone who does predominantly endurance exercise and has a great body? Of course you have! How about people who do predominantly strength exercise? You've seen great bodies on them, too! So it should be clear that you can build a strong, fit, healthy body with different forms of exercise, as long as you perform those exercises properly. In fact, in this chapter, I'm going to show you how you can spend most of your exercise time doing the type you most prefer.

For muscleheads who prefer to spend more time in the weight room, I offer a series of four weightlifting workouts coupled with two cardio workouts. For speed demons who'd rather optimize their time on the road, in the saddle, or on the water, I present a schedule that incorporates just two lifting sessions with four cardio sessions.

Although the actual workouts differ from one another, all of the methods follow sound Metabolism Advantage principles. In the weight room, you'll mix high- and moderate-intensity lifting that targets all of your muscle fiber types. During cardio, you'll focus on high-intensity interval sessions that really rev up your metabolism and keep it going strong, long after your workout ends.

Let's start with the muscleheads. In the following pages, you'll find a program that caters to your strengths.

The Metabolism Advantage Strengthening Program

If you love strengthening exercises, this is your dream program. Rather than having you grind out lots of cardiovascular exercise in your target heart rate zone, this program is based on 4 days of strengthening exercise and just 2 days of short interval workouts.

In two of your workouts, you'll use heavy weights, completing 5 or fewer reps. For these, you'll rest for 2 minutes between exercises and sets. In the other two workouts, you'll use lighter weights, completing 8 to 10 reps. For these high-repetition workouts, you'll alternate between exercises that target opposing muscle groups. For example, for the upper-body high-repetition workout in weeks 1 through 4, you'll do three sets of incline bench presses and lying rows, switching back and forth between exercises for each set. By alternating between opposing muscle groups (called antagonists), you get two benefits. First, by doing a set that targets an antagonist, you'll be stronger on the opposite side when you return to it for the next set. Also, you'll get more of a rest between sets of exercises for the same muscle group. So for this high-repetition workout, you'll need only 1 minute of rest between exercises (and sets).

When sequencing your workouts during the week, split them up to allow at least 48 hours of rest between workouts for each muscle group. For example, you might do the low-repetition, upper-body strengthening workout on Monday, the low-repetition, lower-body workout on Tuesday, an interval workout on Wednesday, the high-repetition, upper-body strengthening workout on Thursday, the higher-repetition, lower-body workout on Friday, and an interval workout on Saturday.

Before and after each workout, warm up and cool down with 5 minutes of light cardio.

STRENGTHENING PROGRAM WEEKS 1–4

■ DAY 1: MONDAY

Upper-Body Low-Repetition Workout	
5-MINUTE LOW-INTENSITY WARMUP:	Cardiovascular bicycling, walking, rowing, or stairclimbing
FLAT BARBELL BENCH PRESS: 1 set of 5 reps, 2 sets of 3 reps, 1 set of 1 rep	Set 1: ___ lb ___ reps Set 2: ___ lb ___ reps Set 3: ___ lb ___ reps Set 4: ___ lb ___ reps
PUSH PRESS: 1 set of 5 reps, 2 sets of 3 reps, 1 set of 1 rep	Set 1: ___ lb ___ reps Set 2: ___ lb ___ reps Set 3: ___ lb ___ reps Set 4: ___ lb ___ reps
PULLUP: 2 sets of 5 reps, 1 set of 3 reps	Set 1: ___ lb ___ reps Set 2: ___ lb ___ reps Set 3: ___ lb ___ reps
DIP: 2 sets of 5 reps, 1 set of 3 reps	Set 1: ___ lb ___ reps Set 2: ___ lb ___ reps Set 3: ___ lb ___ reps
5-MINUTE LOW-INTENSITY COOLDOWN:	Bicycling, walking, rowing, or stairclimbing

■ DAY 2: TUESDAY

Lower-Body Low-Repetition Workout

5-MINUTE LOW-INTENSITY WARMUP:	Bicycling, walking, rowing, or stairclimbing
BARBELL DEADLIFT: 1 set of 5 reps, 2 sets of 3 reps, 1 set of 1 rep	Set 1: ___ lb ___ reps Set 2: ___ lb ___ reps Set 3: ___ lb ___ reps Set 4: ___ lb ___ reps
BARBELL SQUAT: 1 set of 5 reps, 2 sets of 3 reps, 1 set of 1 rep	Set 1: ___ lb ___ reps Set 2: ___ lb ___ reps Set 3: ___ lb ___ reps Set 4: ___ lb ___ reps
BARBELL GOOD MORNING: 2 sets of 5 reps, 1 set of 3 reps	Set 1: ___ lb ___ reps Set 2: ___ lb ___ reps Set 3: ___ lb ___ reps
FRONT SQUAT: 2 sets of 5 reps, 1 set of 3 reps	Set 1: ___ lb ___ reps Set 2: ___ lb ___ reps Set 3: ___ lb ___ reps
5-MINUTE LOW-INTENSITY COOLDOWN:	Bicycling, walking, rowing, or stairclimbing

■ DAY 3: THURSDAY

Upper-Body High-Repetition Workout

5-MINUTE LOW-INTENSITY WARMUP:	Bicycling, walking, rowing, or stairclimbing
UNDERHAND ALTERNATING DUMBBELL INCLINE PRESS: 3 sets of 8–10 reps with each arm	
ALTERNATING DUMBBELL LYING ROW: 3 sets of 8–10 reps with each arm	Press Set 1: ___ lb ___ reps per arm Row Set 1: ___ lb ___ reps per arm Press Set 2: ___ lb ___ reps per arm Row Set 2: ___ lb ___ reps per arm Press Set 3: ___ lb ___ reps per arm Row Set 3: ___ lb ___ reps per arm
SINGLE-ARM BARBELL BICEPS CURL: 3 sets of 8–10 reps with each arm	Set 1 (right arm): ___ lb ___ reps Set 1 (left arm): ___ lb ___ reps Set 2 (right arm): ___ lb ___ reps Set 2 (left arm): ___ lb ___ reps Set 3 (right arm): ___ lb ___ reps Set 3 (left arm): ___ lb ___ reps

PUSHUP ON SWISS BALL: 3 sets of 8–10 reps	Set 1: ___ reps Set 2: ___ reps Set 3: ___ reps
DUMBBELL UPRIGHT ROW: 2 sets of 8–10 reps	
LOW PULLEY ROW: 2 sets of 8–10 reps	Dumbbell Row Set 1: ___ lb ___ reps Pulley Row Set 1: ___ lb ___ reps Dumbbell Row Set 2: ___ lb ___ reps Pulley Row Set 2: ___ lb ___ reps
5-MINUTE LOW-INTENSITY COOLDOWN:	Bicycling, walking, rowing, or stairclimbing

■ DAY 4: FRIDAY

Lower-Body High-Repetition Workout

5-MINUTE LOW-INTENSITY WARMUP:	Bicycling, walking, rowing, or stairclimbing
BULGARIAN SPLIT SQUATS WITH DUMBBELLS: 3 sets of 8–10 reps on each side	
SUITCASE DEADLIFT: 3 sets of 8–10 reps with each arm	Squat Set 1: ___ lb ___ reps per side Deadlift Set 1: ___ lb ___ reps per arm Squat Set 2: ___ lb ___ reps per side Deadlift Set 2: ___ lb ___ reps per arm Squat Set 3: ___ lb ___ reps per side Deadlift Set 3: ___ lb ___ reps per arm
BARBELL SQUAT: 3 sets of 8–10 reps	
LYING LEG CURL: 3 sets of 8–10 reps	Squat Set 1: ___ lb ___ reps Curl Set 1: ___ lb ___ reps Squat Set 2: ___ lb ___ reps Curl Set 2: ___ lb ___ reps Squat Set 3: ___ lb ___ reps Curl Set 3: ___ lb ___ reps
5-MINUTE LOW-INTENSITY COOLDOWN:	Bicycling, walking, rowing, or stairclimbing

STRENGTHENING PROGRAM WEEKS 1–4

Upper-Body Low-Repetition Workout

■ FLAT BARBELL BENCH PRESS
Chest, Shoulders, Triceps

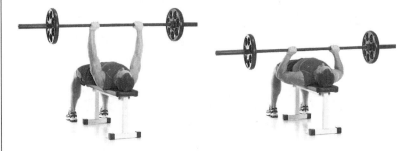

A Lie on a flat bench and position your body so the barbell on the supports is above your face. Grasp the bar with your hands shoulder-width apart. Keep your feet flat on the floor as you lift the weight off the supports and hold the bar above your chest.

B Bend your elbows to the sides as you lower the bar toward your upper chest, stopping when your elbows are in line with your torso.

Pause at the bottom for a second, then press back up. Complete 1 set of 5 reps, 2 sets of 3 reps, and 1 set of 1 rep.

■ PUSH PRESS

Quads, Deltoids, Triceps

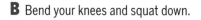

A Grasp a barbell at chest level with an overhand grip, with your hands slightly more than shoulder-width apart.

B Bend your knees and squat down.

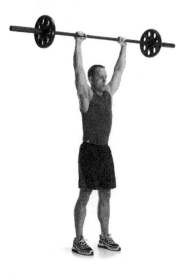

C Explosively straighten your legs as you drive the barbell up, vigorously extending your arms overhead in a shoulder press motion. Lower the barbell to your chest and repeat. Complete 1 set of 5 reps, 2 sets of 3 reps, and 1 set of 1 rep.

■ PULLUP
Upper Back, Biceps, Brachialis

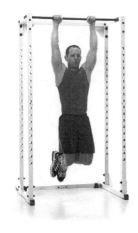

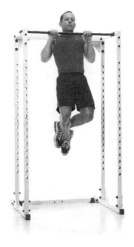

A Hang from an overhead bar with an overhand grip, with your hands shoulder-width apart.

B Pull yourself up until your chin clears the bar.

Lower and repeat, completing 2 sets of 5 reps and 1 set of 3 reps.

NOTE: If you can't pull up your entire body weight, do assisted pullups, either with a partner pushing against your lower back or on a pullup machine that supports some—but not all—of your body weight.

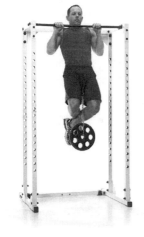

C If you can easily do 5 pullups, either wear a weighted belt or hold a dumbbell between your ankles.

■ DIP
Triceps, Chest

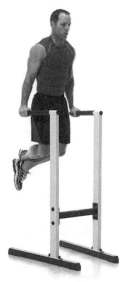

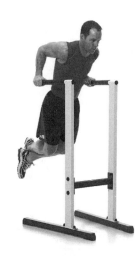

A Depending on your strength, you can do this exercise either on a dip bar with or without weight or on a dip/pullup machine that removes some of the weight from your body. If you need added weight, either use a weighted belt or hold a dumbbell between your ankles.

Mount the dip bar or machine with your palms facing in and your arms extended.

B Keeping your elbows close to your body, bend them and lower your torso until you feel a slight stretch in your shoulders.

Extend your arms and return to the starting position. Complete 2 sets of 5 reps and 1 set of 3 reps.

Lower-Body Low-Repetition Workout

■ BARBELL DEADLIFT
Glutes, Hamstrings, Lower Back

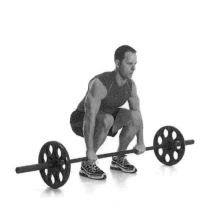

A Place a loaded barbell on the floor and stand with your feet hip-width apart under the center of the bar. Bend your knees, squat down, and grasp the bar with an overhand grip, with your hands shoulder-width or slightly farther apart.

B Keeping your arms and back straight, extend your knees and hips as you lift the bar and stand. As you lift, keep the bar close to your body. Pull your shoulders back at the top of the lift. Complete 1 set of 5 reps, 2 sets of 3 reps, and 1 set of 1 rep.

■ BARBELL SQUAT
Glutes

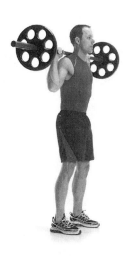

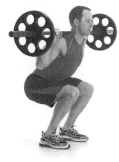

A Position a barbell behind your head, along the backs of your shoulders. Grasp the bar with an overhand grip, your hands slightly wider than shoulder-width apart.

B With your body weight equally distributed between your heels and forefeet, bend your knees and bend forward slightly from the hips until your thighs are parallel to the floor.

Then straighten your legs and rise to the starting position. Throughout, keep your head forward, your back straight, and your feet flat on the floor. Complete 1 set of 5 reps,2 sets of 3 reps, and 1 set of 1 rep.

■ BARBELL GOOD MORNING

Hamstrings, Lower Back

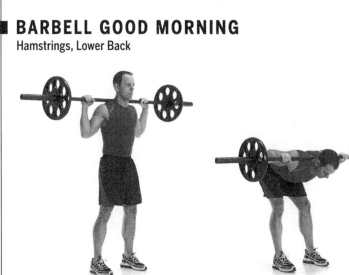

A Position a barbell along the backs of your shoulders, grasping it with an overhand grip, with your hands slightly more than shoulder-width apart.

B Bend forward from the hips, as if you were bowing, but keep your back flat (not rounded). Stop when your torso is parallel to the floor.

Keeping your back and knees extended, return to the starting position. Complete 2 sets of 5 reps and 1 set of 3 reps.

FRONT SQUAT

Glutes

A Use a barbell rack to place a barbell across the fronts of your shoulders at chest height. Cross your arms and place your hands on top of the barbell with your upper arms parallel to the floor. When your your hands are in position, lift the bar from the rack.

B Bend your knees and lower your torso into a squat until your thighs are parallel with the floor.

To rise, extend your knees and hips—pressing equally through your heels and forefeet—until your legs are straight. Throughout, keep your head forward, your back straight, and your feet flat on the floor. Complete 2 sets of 5 reps and 1 set of 3 reps.

Upper-Body High-Repetition Workout

■ UNDERHAND ALTERNATING DUMBBELL INCLINE PRESS
Chest, Shoulders, Triceps

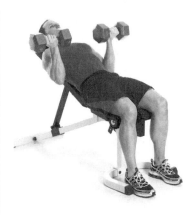 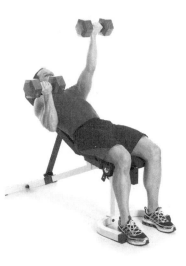

A Sit on an incline bench holding dumbbells in an underhand grip so they rest on your lower thighs. Bring the weights up to your shoulders and lean back against the bench. Position the dumbbells at the sides of your upper chest, with your elbows below the dumbbells.

B Press one dumbbell up until your arm is extended.

Lower the weight to your upper chest and repeat with the other arm. Continue alternating sides until you've completed 8 to 10 reps. Next, do 1 set of Alternating Dumbbell Lying Rows, then another set of Incline Bench Presses. All told, you'll complete 3 sets of each.

ALTERNATING DUMBBELL LYING ROW

Upper Back, Shoulders

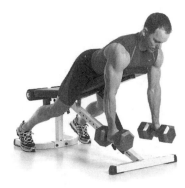 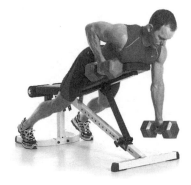

A Lie facedown on a weight bench and grasp a dumbbell in each hand, extending your arms to the floor and letting your shoulders stretch forward. (**NOTE:** The bench should be high enough to let you stretch your shoulders forward without the dumbbells hitting the floor.)

B Pull one dumbbell up, bringing your upper arm just beyond horizontal.

Lower and repeat with the other arm. Continue alternating sides for 8 to 10 reps on each side. Alternate this exercise with Underhand Alternating Dumbbell Incline Presses, continuing until you've completed 3 sets of each.

■ SINGLE-ARM BARBELL BICEPS CURL

Biceps

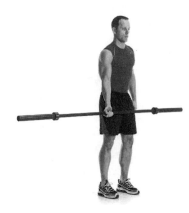 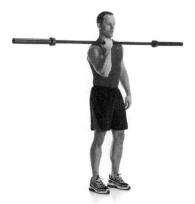

A Grasp either a long or short barbell (depending on your strength) with your right hand, holding the center of the bar with an under-hand grip.

B Keeping your right elbow close to your side, raise the bar until your right forearm is vertical.

Then lower it until your arm is fully extended. Complete 8 to 10 reps, then repeat with your left arm. Alternate this exercise with Pushups on Swiss Ball, continuing until you've completed 3 sets of each.

PUSHUP ON SWISS BALL

Chest

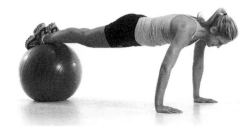

A Kneel with your belly on a Swiss ball. Roll forward until you are in a plank position, with your hands on the floor under your chest and your feet on the ball.

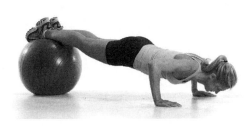

B Keeping your back straight, bend your elbows and lower your chest to the floor.

Extend your arms to return to the starting position. Complete 8 to 10 reps. Alternate this exercise with Single-Arm Barbell Biceps Curls, continuing until you've completed 3 sets of each.

■ DUMBBELL UPRIGHT ROW

Deltoids

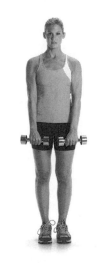 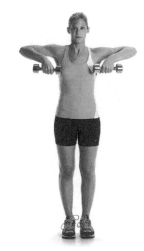

A Grasp a pair of dumbbells with your arms extended down in front of your body and your palms facing the fronts of your thighs.

B Pull the dumbbells up the centerline of your body, bending your elbows out to the sides. Allow your wrists to flex as you raise the weights, but don't shrug your shoulders.

Lower and repeat, completing 8 to 10 reps. Alternate this exercise with Low Pulley Rows, continuing until you've completed 2 sets of each.

LOW PULLEY ROW

Back

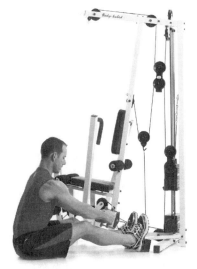 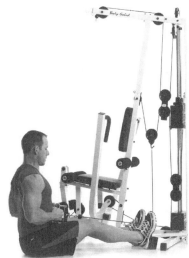

A Sit on the seated row platform with your knees bent. Grasp the cable attachment and push back slightly to extend your legs until there's just a slight bend in your knees. Lean forward slightly from your hips.

B Bend your elbows as you pull the cable attachment to your waist and sit upright. Pull your shoulders back and push your chest forward.

Return to the starting position and repeat 8 to 10 times. Alternate this exercise with Dumbbell Upright Rows, continuing until you've completed 2 sets of each.

Lower-Body High-Repetition Workout

■ BULGARIAN SPLIT SQUATS WITH DUMBBELLS

Quads, Hamstrings, Glutes

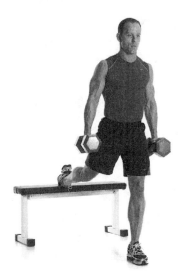
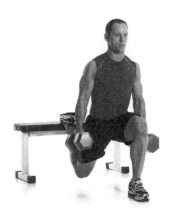

A Stand with your back to an exercise bench and grasp a dumbbell in each hand, placing your hands at your hips. Place the instep of one foot on the bench, supporting your weight with the other foot.

B Keeping your torso as straight as possible, bend both knees until your front leg forms a 90-degree angle.

Pause, then press back up. Complete 8 to 10 reps. Alternate this exercise with Suitcase Deadlifts, continuing until you've completed 3 sets of each.

■ SUITCASE DEADLIFT
Glutes, Hamstrings, Quads, Core Muscles

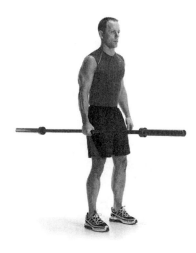

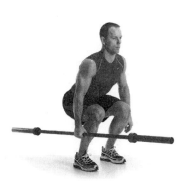

A Grasp a barbell in the center with your right hand and hold it at your right side as if it were a heavy suitcase.

B Bend your knees and squat down as if you were trying to place your suitcase on the floor.

Keeping your arms and back straight, extend your knees and hips and return to the starting position. Complete 8 to 10 reps with each arm. Alternate this exercise with Bulgarian Split Squats, continuing until you've completed 3 sets of each.

BARBELL HACK SQUAT

Quads, Glutes, Hamstrings

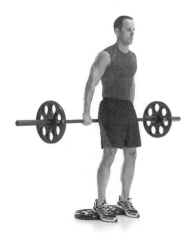

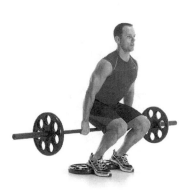

A Set a 25-pound weight plate about a foot behind each support of a squat rack. Set a barbell on the rack at about hip level and stand with your back to it, then grasp it with a shoulder-width grip behind your back. Next, slowly walk backward toward the weight plates until both your heels are elevated on them.

B Keeping your back as straight as possible, bend your knees and squat down as far as you can.

When you've reached your lowest point, push your feet into the floor to rise to the starting position. Complete 8 to 10 reps. Alternate this exercise with Lying Leg Curls, continuing until you've completed 3 sets of each.

■ LYING LEG CURL

Hamstrings

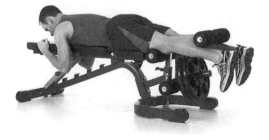

A Lie facedown on the hamstring curl machine with your knees just beyond the edge of the bench and your legs under the lever pads. Grasp the handles for support.

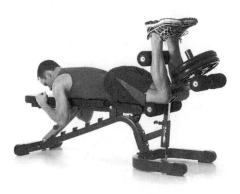

B Bend your knees and raise the pads toward the backs of your thighs.

Then reverse the motion, lowering the pads until your knees are straight. Repeat 8 to 10 times. Alternate this exercise with Barbell Hack Squats, continuing until you've completed 3 sets of each.

STRENGTHENING PROGRAM WEEKS 5–8

■ DAY 1: MONDAY

Upper-Body Low-Repetition Workout

5-MINUTE LOW-INTENSITY WARMUP:	Bicycling, walking, rowing, or stairclimbing

BENT-OVER BARBELL ROW: 1 set of 5 reps, 2 sets of 3 reps, 1 set of 1 rep	Set 1: ___ lb ___ reps Set 2: ___ lb ___ reps Set 3: ___ lb ___ reps Set 4: ___ lb ___ reps
OVERHAND ALTERNATING DUMBBELL INCLINE PRESS: 1 set of 5 reps, 2 sets of 3 reps, 1 set of 1 rep	Set 1: ___ lb ___ reps Set 2: ___ lb ___ reps Set 3: ___ lb ___ reps Set 4: ___ lb ___ reps
ALTERNATING DUMBBELL SHOULDER PRESS ON SWISS BALL: 2 sets of 5 reps with each arm, 1 set of 3 reps with each arm	Set 1: ___ lb ___ reps Set 2: ___ lb ___ reps Set 3 ___ lb ___ reps
BARBELL CLEAN: 2 sets of 5 reps, 1 set of 3 reps	Set 1: ___ lb ___ reps Set 2: ___ lb ___ reps Set 3 ___ lb ___ reps
5-MINUTE LOW-INTENSITY COOLDOWN:	Bicycling, walking, rowing, or stairclimbing

■ DAY 2: TUESDAY

Lower-Body Low-Repetition Workout

5-MINUTE LOW-INTENSITY WARMUP:	Bicycling, walking, rowing, or stairclimbing

BARBELL HACK SQUAT: 1 set of 5 reps, 2 sets of 3 reps, 1 set of 1 rep	Set 1: ___ lb ___ reps Set 2: ___ lb ___ reps Set 3: ___ lb ___ reps Set 4: ___ lb ___ reps
BARBELL GOOD MORNING: 1 set of 5 reps, 2 sets of 3 reps, 1 set of 1 rep	Set 1: ___ lb ___ reps Set 2: ___ lb ___ reps Set 3: ___ lb ___ reps Set 4: ___ lb ___ reps

OVERHEAD DUMBBELL SQUAT: 2 sets of 5 reps, 1 set of 3 reps	Set 1: ___ lb ___ reps Set 2: ___ lb ___ reps Set 3: ___ lb ___ reps
STIFF-LEG DEADLIFT WITH DUMBBELLS: 2 sets of 5 reps, 1 set of 3 reps	Set 1: ___ lb ___ reps Set 2: ___ lb ___ reps Set 3: ___ lb ___ reps
5-MINUTE LOW-INTENSITY COOLDOWN:	Bicycling, walking, rowing, or stairclimbing

■ DAY 3: THURSDAY

Upper-Body High-Repetition Workout

5-MINUTE LOW-INTENSITY WARMUP:	Bicycling, walking, rowing, or stairclimbing
CHINUP: 3 sets of 8–10 reps	
FLAT BARBELL BENCH PRESS: 3 sets of 8–10 reps	Chinup Set 1: ___ lb ___ reps Press Set 1: ___ lb ___ reps Chinup Set 2: ___ lb ___ reps Press Set 2: ___ lb ___ reps Chinup Set 3: ___ lb ___ reps Press Set 3: ___ lb ___ reps
DIP: 3 sets of 8–10 reps	
ALTERNATING DUMBBELL CURL ON SWISS BALL: 3 sets of 8–10 reps with each arm	Dip Set 1: ___ lb ___ reps Curl Set 1: ___ lb ___ reps per arm Dip Set 2: ___ lb ___ reps Curl Set 2: ___ lb ___ reps per arm Dip Set 3: ___ lb ___ reps Curl Set 3: ___ lb ___ reps per arm
SIDE RAISE: 2 sets of 8–10 reps	
BARBELL OVERHEAD PRESS: 2 sets of 8–10 reps	Raise Set 1: ___ lb ___ reps Press Set 1: ___ lb ___ reps Raise Set 2: ___ lb ___ reps Press Set 2: ___ lb ___ reps
5-MINUTE LOW-INTENSITY COOLDOWN:	Bicycling, walking, rowing, or stairclimbing

■ DAY 4: FRIDAY

Lower-Body High-Repetition Workout	
5-MINUTE LOW-INTENSITY WARMUP:	Bicycling, walking, rowing, or stairclimbing
LEG PRESS: 3 sets of 8–10 reps on each side	
LYING LEG CURL: 3 sets of 8–10 reps	Press Set 1: ___ lb ___ reps Curl Set 1: ___ lb ___ reps Press Set 2: ___ lb ___ reps Curl Set 2: ___ lb ___ reps Press Set 3: ___ lb ___ reps Curl Set 3: ___ lb ___ reps
DUMBBELL OVERHEAD WALKING LUNGE: 3 sets of 8–10 reps on each side	
SWISS BALL HYPEREXTENSION: 3 sets of 8–10 reps	Lunge Set 1: ___ lb ___ reps per side Hyperextension Set 1: ___ lb ___ reps Lunge Set 2: ___ lb ___ reps per side Hyperextension Set 2: ___ lb ___ reps Lunge Set 3: ___ lb ___ reps per side Hyperextension Set 3: ___ lb ___ reps
5-MINUTE LOW-INTENSITY COOLDOWN:	Bicycling, walking, rowing, or stairclimbing

Upper-Body Low-Repetition Workout

■ BENT-OVER BARBELL ROW
Upper and Lower Back, Biceps

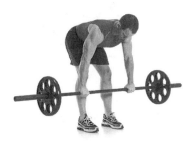 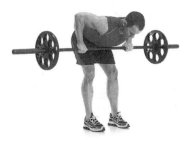

A Bend your knees slightly and bend forward with your back straight. Grasp a loaded barbell with an overhand grip, with your hands slightly more than shoulder–width apart.

B Bend your elbows, bringing them toward the ceiling as you pull the bar toward your midsection.

Extend your arms to the starting position, allowing your shoulders to stretch forward slightly. Complete 1 set of 5 reps, 2 sets of 3 reps, and 1 set of 1 rep.

■ ALTERNATING DUMBBELL INCLINE PRESS

Chest, Shoulders, Triceps

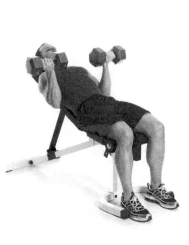 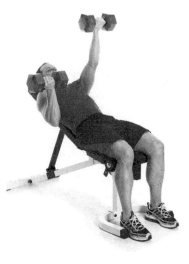

A Sit on an incline bench holding dumbbells in an underhand grip so they rest on your lower thighs. Bring the weights up to your shoulders and lean back against the bench. Position the dumbbells at the sides of your upper chest, with your elbows below the dumbbells.

B Press one dumbbell up with your elbow to the side until your arm is extended. Lower the weight to your upper chest and repeat with the other arm. Complete 1 set of 5 reps, 2 sets of 3 reps, and 1 set of 1 rep.

ALTERNATING DUMBBELL SHOULDER PRESS ON SWISS BALL

Deltoids, Triceps

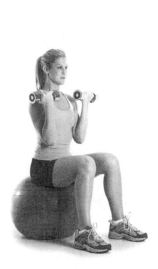 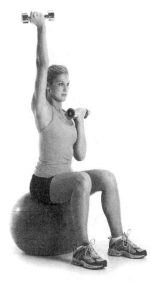

A Sit on a Swiss ball with your knees bent and your feet flat on the floor. Hold a dumbbell with an underhand grip next to each shoulder, with your elbows under your wrists and your palms facing in.

B Press one dumbbell up until that arm is extended overhead. Lower and repeat with the other arm. Complete 2 sets of 5 reps and 1 set of 3 reps.

■ BARBELL CLEAN

Hips, Shoulders, Legs, Upper Back

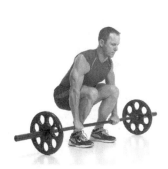

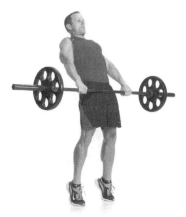

A Place a loaded barbell on the floor and stand with your feet slightly more than hip-width apart just under the bar. Squat down and grasp the bar with an overhand grip, with your hands slightly more than shoulder-width apart. With your back arched slightly, position your shoulders over the bar.

B Extend your knees and hips as you lift the bar, at first keeping your arms extended.

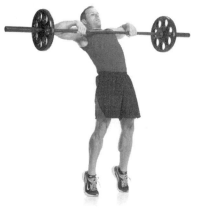

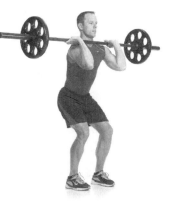

C Once the bar reaches your knees, vigorously raise your shoulders and pull the barbell up as you flex your elbows out to the sides in an upright rowing motion. Keep the bar close to your body the entire time, then catch it at the top position. Lower and repeat. Complete 2 sets of 5 reps and 1 set of 3 reps.

Lower-Body Low-Repetition Workout

■ BARBELL HACK SQUAT
Quads, Glutes, Hamstrings

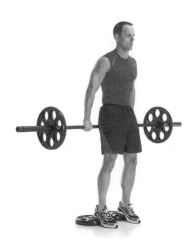 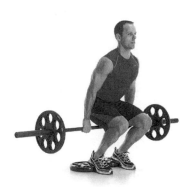

A Set a 25-pound weight plate about a foot behind each support of a squat rack. Set a barbell on the rack at about hip level and stand with your back to it, then grasp it with a shoulder-width grip behind your back. Next, slowly walk backward toward the weight plates until both your heels are elevated on them.

B Keeping your back as straight as possible, bend your knees and squat down as far as you can.

When you've reached your lowest point, push your feet into the floor to rise to the starting position. Complete 1 set of 5 reps, 2 sets of 3 reps, and 1 set of 1 rep.

■ BARBELL GOOD MORNING

Hamstrings, Lower Back

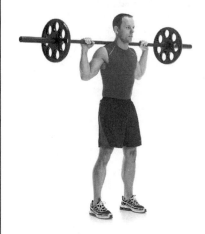 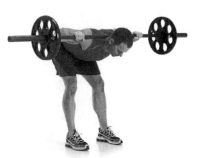

A Position a barbell along the backs of your shoulders, grasping it with an overhand grip, with your hands slightly more than shoulder-width apart.

B Bend forward from the hips, as if you were bowing, but keep your back flat (not rounded). Stop when your torso is parallel to the floor.

Keeping your back and knees extended, return to the starting position. Complete 1 set of 5 reps, 2 sets of 3 reps, and 1 set of 1 rep.

■ OVERHEAD DUMBBELL SQUAT

Quads, Glutes, Core Muscles

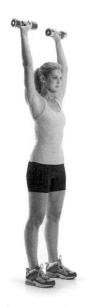

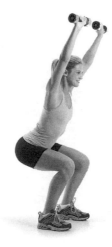

A Grasp a dumbbell in each hand and extend your arms overhead.

B Bend your knees and lower your torso until your thighs are parallel to the floor.

Then extend your knees and hips and stand up. Keep your head forward, your back straight, and your chest high. Complete 2 sets of 5 reps and 1 set of 3 reps.

■ STIFF-LEG DEADLIFT WITH DUMBBELLS

Upper and Lower Back, Glutes, Hamstrings

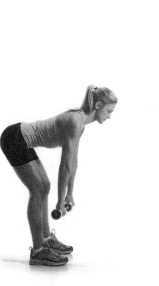 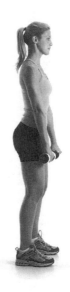

A Stand with your feet shoulder-width apart, holding a pair of dumbbells at thigh level with an overhand grip, with your hands shoulder-width apart. With your knees slightly bent, bend forward from the hips, lowering the dumbbells toward your feet until you feel a mild stretch in your hamstrings.

B With your knees bent, lift the dumbbells as you stand upright. Complete 2 sets of 5 reps and 1 set of 3 reps.

Upper-Body High-Repetition Workout

■ CHINUP
Upper Back, Biceps

You can do chinups wearing a weighted a belt or with a dumbbell between your feet, assisted by a partner, or on a chinup machine.

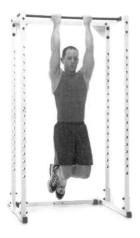 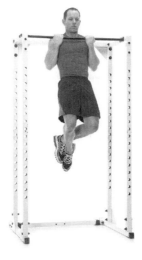

A To do a basic chinup, hang from an overhead bar with an underhand grip, with your hands shoulder-width apart.

B Extend your chest and pull yourself up until your chin clears the bar or your chest touches it.

Lower and repeat. Complete 8 to 10 reps. Alternate this exercise with Flat Barbell Bench Presses, continuing until you've completed 3 sets of each.

■ FLAT BARBELL BENCH PRESS

Chest, Shoulders, Triceps

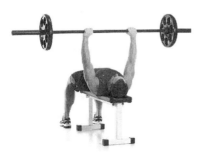

A Lie on a flat bench and position your body so the barbell on the supports is above your face. Grasp the bar with your hands shoulder-width apart. Keep your feet flat on the floor as you lift the weight off the supports and hold the bar above your chest.

B Bend your elbows out to the sides as you lower the bar to your upper chest, stopping when your elbows are in line with your torso.

Pause at the bottom for a second and press back up. Complete 8 to 10 reps. Alternate this exercise with Chinups, continuing until you've completed 3 sets of each.

■ DIP

Triceps, Chest

Depending on your strength, you can do this exercise either on a dip bar with or without weight or on a dip/pullup machine that removes some of the weight from your body. If you need added weight, either use a weighted belt or hold a dumbbell between your ankles.

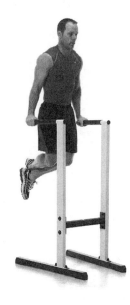 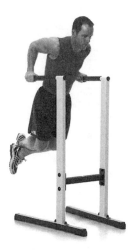

A Mount the dip bar or machine with your palms facing in and your arms extended.

B Keeping your elbows close to your body, bend them and lower your torso until you feel a slight stretch in your shoulders.

Extend your arms and return to the starting position. Complete 8 to 10 reps. Alternate this exercise with Alternating Dumbbell Curls on Swiss Ball, continuing until you've completed 3 sets of each.

■ ALTERNATING DUMBBELL CURL ON SWISS BALL

Biceps

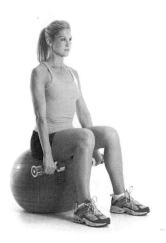
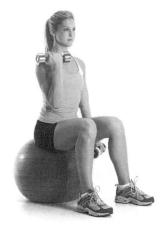

A Sit on a Swiss ball with your knees bent and your feet flat on the floor. Hold a dumbbell in an overhand grip at each side, with your palms facing in and your arms straight.

B Keeping your elbows close to your sides, raise one dumbbell, rotating your forearm until it is vertical and your palm faces your shoulder.

Lower to the starting position and repeat with the opposite arm. Continue to alternate left and right until you've completed 8 to 10 reps on each side. Alternate this exercise with Dips, continuing until you've completed 3 sets of each.

■ SIDE RAISE
Deltoids

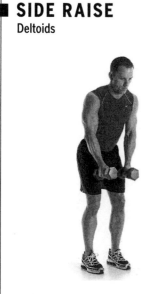 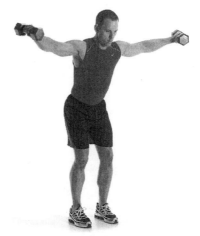

A Holding a pair of dumbbells in front of your thighs, bend forward from your hips with your knees slightly bent.

B With your elbows slightly bent, raise your arms out to the sides until your elbows reach shoulder height.

Lower and repeat. Complete 8 to 10 reps. Alternate this exercise with Barbell Overhead Presses, continuing until you've completed 2 sets of each.

■ BARBELL OVERHEAD PRESS

Shoulders, Trapezius, Triceps

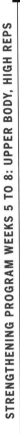

A Take a barbell off the supports of a squat rack and hold it at collarbone level with an overhand grip, with your hands shoulder-width apart.

B Walk back a step or two and then, with your knees slightly bent, press the bar overhead until your arms are straight.

Lower the bar to chin level and repeat. Complete 8 to 10 reps. Alternate this exercise with Side Raises, continuing until you've completed 3 sets of each.

Lower-Body High-Repetition Workout

■ LEG PRESS
Quads

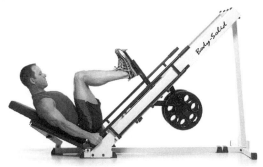

A Sit on a leg press machine with your back against the padded support. Place your feet on the platform and grasp the handles at your sides for support.

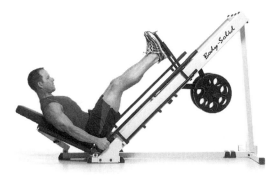

B Extend your knees and hips to push the platform away from you.

Bend your knees to return to the starting position. Keep your knees pointed up; don't let them splay outward. Also, don't allow your heels to rise off the platform. Complete 8 to 10 reps. Alternate this exercise with Lying Leg Curls, continuing until you've completed 3 sets of each.

■ LYING LEG CURL

Hamstrings

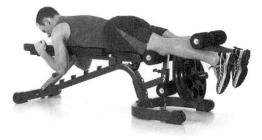

A Lie facedown on the hamstring curl machine with your knees just beyond the edge of the bench and your legs under the lever pads. Grasp the handles for support.

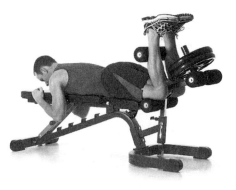

B Bend your knees and raise the pads toward the backs of your thighs.

Then reverse the motion, lowering the pads until your knees are straight. Repeat 8 to 10 times. Alternate this exercise with Leg Presses, continuing until you've completed 3 sets of each.

■ DUMBBELL OVERHEAD WALKING LUNGE

Glutes, Quads, Hamstrings, Core Muscles

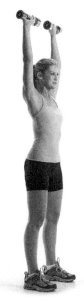

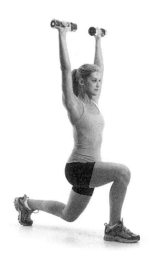

A Grasp a dumbbell in each hand and extend your arms overhead.

B Lunge forward with your right leg, landing on your heel and then your forefoot. Lower your body by bending your knees until they both form right angles and the knee of your left leg is almost in contact with the floor.

Step forward with your left leg, landing on your heel and then your forefoot. Continue lunging forward until you've completed 8 to 10 repetitions on each side. Alternate this exercise with Swiss Ball Hyperextensions, continuing until you've completed 3 sets of each.

■ SWISS BALL HYPEREXTENSIONS

Lower Back

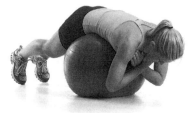

A Lie facedown on a Swiss ball with your legs straight and your torso rounded over the ball.

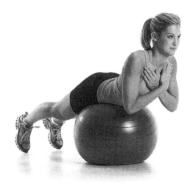

B With your hands folded over your chest, extend your spine and lift your chest off the ball. Complete 8 to 10 reps. Alternate this exercise with Dumbbell Overhead Walking Lunges, continuing until you've completed 3 sets of each.

STRENGTH-FOCUSED CARDIO

On the strength-focused plan, you'll do just two cardio workouts a week. Do any form of cardio you like, whether running, cycling, rowing, or something else. These workouts remain the same for all 8 weeks.

INTERVAL WORKOUT #1

    5-minute low-intensity warmup
    Intervals: 90 seconds at high intensity, 180 seconds at low intensity
    Perform 4 total intervals
    5-minute low-intensity cooldown

INTERVAL WORKOUT #2

    5-minute low-intensity warmup
    Intervals: 30 seconds at high intensity, 30 seconds at low intensity
    Perform 15 total intervals
    5-minute low-intensity cooldown

YOUR STRENGTH-FOCUSED SCHEDULE

Now that you have the moves to help you maximize strength, let's talk about what to do with them. The following sequence includes four strength workouts, two interval workouts, and one low-intensity cardio day. It allows you to maximize your time in the gym and provides 2 days off.

In Chapters 5 and 8, I scheduled your workouts in such a way that you never did your intense cardio on the same day as your weight-training workouts. Splitting up your sessions in that way required you to work out 6 days a week.

This strength-centered schedule provides an additional off day. There is a downside, however, to having more sedentary days each week. Although I can't cite a study to prove it, I can tell you from experience that the more days a week you train, the better your results. Remember the afterburn, the metabolism boost you get after a workout as your body repairs your muscles? Well, you'll want that afterburn after every workout, every day, to increase your Metabolism Advantage power.

For every problem, however, there's a solution. You'll make up for your extra days off by adding low-intensity cardio to your schedule. For this, you just need to move. Go for a walk with your spouse, play actively with your kids or dog, or cut the grass with a push mower. You're limited only by your own creativity. Just be sure that you do some form of physical activity. It all counts.

Use this schedule.

MONDAY: Upper-body low-repetition strengthening workout
TUESDAY: Lower-body low-repetition strengthening workout in the morning; interval cardio in the evening
WEDNESDAY: 30 minutes of low-intensity cardio
THURSDAY: Upper-body high-repetition strengthening workout
FRIDAY: Lower-body high-repetition strengthening workout in the morning; interval cardio workout in the evening
SATURDAY: Off
SUNDAY: Off

The Metabolism Advantage Endurance Program

If you love cardio, this is your dream program. You can spend most of your time on the pavement or in the saddle, with 4 days of interval work and only 2 days of total-body strengthening workouts.

Because you'll hit the weight room just twice a week, you can focus on high-resistance, low-repetition workouts and not worry about putting too much stress on your nervous system. You don't need to do one high-intensity session and one moderate-intensity session as I've recommended for other approaches.

When scheduling workouts each week, space your total-body workouts at least 48 hours apart. For example, you might do an interval workout on Monday, a total-body workout on Tuesday, an interval session on Wednesday, a total-body workout on Thursday, an interval session on Friday, and an interval session on Saturday.

In the weight room, rest for 1 to $1\frac{1}{2}$ minutes between sets. Warm up before your weight room workouts with 5 minutes of light cardio and cool down after all workouts with 5 minutes of light cardio.

ENDURANCE-FOCUSED CARDIO

On this plan, you'll complete four interval workouts a week. Do any form of cardio that you like, whether running, cycling, rowing, or stairclimbing. These workouts are the same for all 8 weeks.

INTERVAL WORKOUT #1
5-minute low-intensity warmup
Intervals: 30 seconds at high intensity, 90 seconds at low
    intensity
Perform 10 total intervals
5-minute low-intensity cooldown

INTERVAL WORKOUT #2
5-minute low-intensity warmup
Intervals: 60 seconds at high intensity, 60 seconds at low
    intensity
Perform 15 total intervals
5-minute low-intensity walking cooldown

INTERVAL WORKOUT #3
5-minute low-intensity warmup
Intervals: 90 seconds at high intensity, 180 seconds at low
    intensity
Perform 7 total intervals
5-minute low-intensity cooldown

INTERVAL WORKOUT #4

5-minute low-intensity warmup

Intervals: 30 seconds at high intensity, 30 seconds at low
intensity

Perform 30 total intervals

5-minute low-intensity stepping cooldown

ENDURANCE-FOCUSED WEIGHT WORKOUTS: WEEKS 1–4

■ DAY 1

5-MINUTE LOW-INTENSITY WARMUP:	Bicycling, walking, rowing, or stairclimbing
DUMBBELL SQUAT: 3 sets of 5–7 reps (1 set with weights at chest, 1 set with weights extended forward, 1 set with weights overhead)	Set 1 (weights at chest): ___ lb ___ reps Set 2 (weights extended forward): ___ lb ___ reps Set 3 (weights overhead): ___ lb ___ reps
ALTERNATING FLAT DUMBBELL BENCH PRESS: 3 sets of 5–7 reps with each arm	Set 1: ___ lb ___ reps per arm Set 2: ___ lb ___ reps per arm Set 3: ___ lb ___ reps per arm
DUMBBELL WALKING LUNGE: 3 sets of 5–7 reps on each side	Set 1: ___ lb ___ reps per side Set 2: ___ lb ___ reps per side Set 3: ___ lb ___ reps per side
ALTERNATING DUMBBELL SHOULDER PRESS ON SWISS BALL: 3 sets of 5–7 reps with each arm	Set 1: ___ lb ___ reps per arm Set 2: ___ lb ___ reps per arm Set 3: ___ lb ___ reps per arm
DIP: 3 sets of 5–7 reps	Set 1: ___ lb ___ reps Set 2: ___ lb ___ reps Set 3: ___ lb ___ reps
5-MINUTE LOW-INTENSITY COOLDOWN:	Bicycling, walking, rowing, or stairclimbing

DAY 2

5-MINUTE LOW-INTENSITY WARMUP:	Bicycling, walking, rowing, or stairclimbing
BARBELL DEADLIFT: 3 sets of 5–7 reps	Set 1: ___ lb ___ reps Set 2: ___ lb ___ reps Set 3: ___ lb ___ reps
PULLUP: 3 sets of 5–7 reps (1 set with wide overhand grip; 1 set with neutral grip; 1 set with narrow underhand grip)	Set 1 (wide overhand grip): ___ lb ___ reps Set 2 (neutral grip): ___ lb ___ reps Set 3 (narrow underhand grip): ___ lb ___ reps
SINGLE-LEG SWISS BALL LEG CURL: 3 sets of 5–7 reps with each leg	Set 1 (right leg): ___ reps Set 1 (left leg): ___ reps Set 2 (right leg): ___ reps Set 2 (left leg): ___ reps Set 3 (right leg): ___ reps Set 3 (left leg): ___ reps
ALTERNATING DUMBBELL CURL: 3 sets of 5–7 reps with each arm (1 set with underhand grip, 1 set with overhand grip, 1 set with neutral grip)	Set 1 (underhand grip): ___ lb ___ reps per arm Set 2 (overhand grip): ___ lb ___ reps per arm Set 3 (neutral grip): ___ lb ___ reps per arm
BARBELL ROLLOUT: 3 sets of 5–7 reps	Set 1: ___ lb ___ reps Set 2: ___ lb ___ reps Set 3: ___ lb ___ reps
5-MINUTE LOW-INTENSITY COOLDOWN:	Bicycling, walking, rowing, or stairclimbing

Total-Body Workout #1

■ DUMBBELL SQUAT
Quads, Glutes, Hamstrings

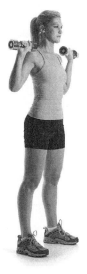

A Standing with your body weight equally distributed between your heels and your forefeet, grasp a pair of dumbbells at chest level.

B Bend your knees and lower your torso until your thighs are parallel to the floor. Keep your head forward, your back straight, and your feet flat on the floor. Extend your knees and hips and rise until your legs are straight. Complete 1 set of 5 to 7 reps. Repeat, this time holding the dumbbells with your arms extended in front of you, for 5 to 7 reps. Then repeat while holding the dumbbells overhead for 5 to 7 reps.

■ ALTERNATING FLAT DUMBBELL BENCH PRESS

Chest, Shoulders, Triceps

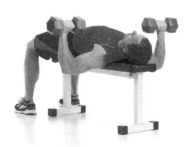 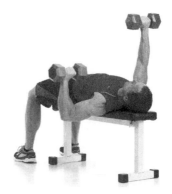

A Lie on a weight bench. Grasp a pair of dumbbells with an overhand grip, with your elbows bent and your hands at the sides of your chest.

B Press one dumbbell up, extending your arm and keeping the dumbbell above your nipple.

Lower and repeat with the other arm. Continue alternating sides until you've completed 5 to 7 reps. Complete 3 sets.

■ DUMBBELL WALKING LUNGE

Glutes, Hamstrings, Quads

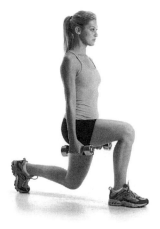

A Holding a pair of dumbbells at your sides, lunge forward with your right leg, landing on your heel and then your forefoot. Lower your body by bending your knees until they both form right angles and the knee of your left leg is almost in contact with the floor.

B Step forward with your left leg, landing on your heel and then your forefoot. Continue lunging forward until you've completed 5 to 7 repetitions on each side. Complete 3 sets.

ALTERNATING DUMBBELL SHOULDER PRESS ON SWISS BALL

Deltoids, Triceps

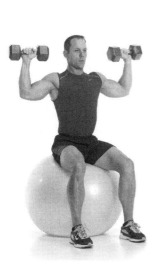 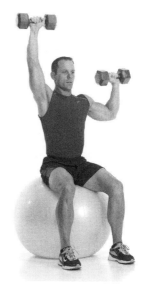

A Sit on a Swiss ball with your knees bent and your feet flat on the floor. Hold a dumbbell with an overhand grip next to each shoulder, with your elbows under your wrists and your palms facing forward.

B Press one dumbbell up until that arm is extended overhead.

Lower and repeat with the other arm. Complete 3 sets of 5 to 7 reps with each arm.

DIP

Triceps, Chest

Depending on your strength, you can do this exercise either on a dip bar with or without weight or on a dip/pullup machine that removes some of the weight from your body. If you need added weight, either use a weighted belt or hold a dumbbell between your ankles.

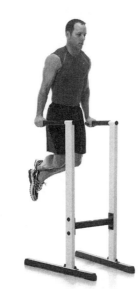 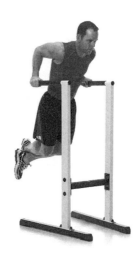

A Mount the dip bar or machine with your palms facing in and your arms extended.

B Keeping your elbows close to your body, bend them and lower your torso until you feel a slight stretch in your shoulders. Extend your arms and return to the starting position. Complete 3 sets of 5 to 7 reps each.

Total-Body Workout #2

■ BARBELL DEADLIFT
Glutes, Hamstrings, Lower Back

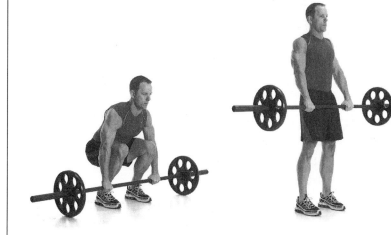

A Place a loaded barbell on the floor and stand with your feet hip-width apart under the center of the bar. Bend your knees, squat down, and grasp the bar with an overhand grip, with your hands shoulder-width or slightly farther apart.

B Keeping your arms and back straight, extend your knees and hips as you lift the bar and stand. As you lift, keep the bar close to your body. Pull your shoulders back at the top of the lift. Complete 3 sets of 5 to 7 reps.

■ PULLUP
Upper Back, Biceps, Brachialis

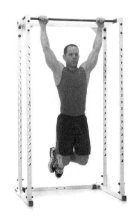

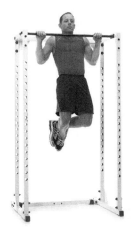

A Hang from an overhead bar with an overhand grip, with your hands slightly more than shoulder-width apart.

B Pull yourself up until your chin clears the bar. Lower and repeat for 5 to 7 reps.

NOTE: If you can't pull up your entire weight, do assisted pullups, either with a partner pushing against your lower back or on a pullup machine that supports some—but not all—of your body weight. If you can easily do 5 to 7 reps, either wear a weighted belt or hold a dumbbell between your ankles.

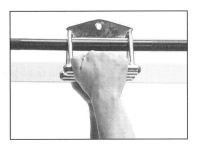

C For your next set, hook a low pulley row attachment over the overhead bar so that you can pull up using a parallel (palms facing each other) grip.

D For your last set, space your hands less than shoulder-width apart (in a narrow grip) and use an underhand grip.

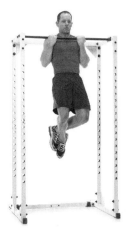

■ SINGLE-LEG SWISS BALL LEG CURL

Hamstrings, Glutes

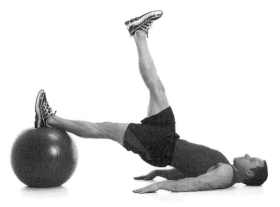

A Lie on your back with your heels and lower calves on a Swiss ball. Lift your hips until your body forms an incline. Lift your right leg into the air, balancing your body weight with just your left leg against the ball.

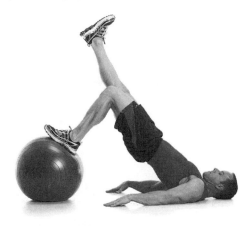

B Bend your left knee and pull the ball toward you.

Pause for a second, then slowly reverse the sequence. Complete 5 to 7 reps and then repeat with the other leg. Complete 3 sets.

■ ALTERNATING DUMBBELL CURL
Biceps

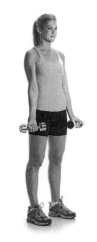

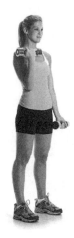

A Stand holding a pair of dumbbells at your sides with an underhand grip, your palms facing forward, and your arms straight.

B Keeping your elbows close to your sides, raise one dumbbell.

Lower to the starting position and repeat with the other arm. Continue to alternate sides, completing 5 to 7 reps with each arm.

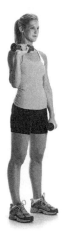

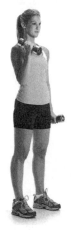

C For your next set, hold the dumbbells with an overhand grip so your palms are facing backward, lifting the backs of your hands toward your shoulders.

D For your last set, use a neutral grip, with your palms facing inward.

BARBELL ROLLOUT
Abdominals, Lower Back, Shoulders

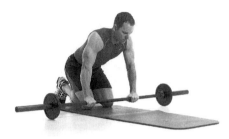

A Kneel on an exercise mat behind a barbell with a 5-pound plate at each end. Grasp the bar with your hands shoulder-width apart and directly beneath your shoulders.

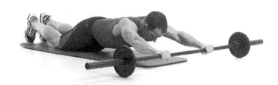

B Slowly allow the bar to roll out and let your body to travel with it. Let your arms extend forward over your head and lower your face as close as possible to the floor without rounding your back.

When you've reached your farthest point, use your core muscles to return to the starting position. Complete 3 sets of 5 to 7 reps.

ENDURANCE-FOCUSED WEIGHT WORKOUTS:
WEEKS 5–8

◼ DAY 1

5-MINUTE LOW-INTENSITY WARMUP:	Bicycling, walking, rowing, or stairclimbing
BARBELL DEADLIFT: 3 sets of 4–6 reps	Set 1: ___ lb ___ reps Set 2: ___ lb ___ reps Set 3: ___ lb ___ reps
FLAT BARBELL BENCH PRESS: 3 sets of 4–6 reps	Set 1: ___ lb ___ reps Set 2: ___ lb ___ reps Set 3: ___ lb ___ reps
STEPUP: 3 sets of 4–6 reps on each side	Set 1: ___ lb ___ reps per side Set 2: ___ lb ___ reps per side Set 3: ___ lb ___ reps per side
OVERHEAD BARBELL SHOULDER PRESS: 3 sets of 5–7 reps	Set 1: ___ lb ___ reps Set 2: ___ lb ___ reps Set 3: ___ lb ___ reps
PULLUP: 3 sets of 5–7 reps	Set 1: ___ lb ___ reps Set 2: ___ lb ___ reps Set 3: ___ lb ___ reps
5-MINUTE LOW-INTENSITY COOLDOWN:	Bicycling, walking, rowing, or stairclimbing

DAY 2

5-MINUTE LOW-INTENSITY WARMUP:	Bicycling, walking, rowing, or stairclimbing	
BARBELL SQUAT: 3 sets of 4–6 reps	Set 1: ___ lb	___ reps
	Set 2: ___ lb	___ reps
	Set 3: ___ lb	___ reps
DIP: 3 sets of 4–6 reps	Set 1: ___ lb	___ reps
	Set 2: ___ lb	___ reps
	Set 3: ___ lb	___ reps
BARBELL GOOD MORNING: 3 sets of 4–6 reps	Set 1: ___ lb	___ reps
	Set 2: ___ lb	___ reps
	Set 3: ___ lb	___ reps
BARBELL CURL: 3 sets of 4–6 reps	Set 1: ___ lb	___ reps
	Set 2: ___ lb	___ reps
	Set 3: ___ lb	___ reps
BARBELL ROLLOUT: 3 sets of 5–7 reps	Set 1: ___ lb	___ reps
	Set 2: ___ lb	___ reps
	Set 3: ___ lb	___ reps
5-MINUTE LOW-INTENSITY COOLDOWN:	Bicycling, walking, rowing, or stairclimbing	

Total-Body Workout #1

■ **BARBELL DEADLIFT**
Glutes, Hamstrings, Lower Back

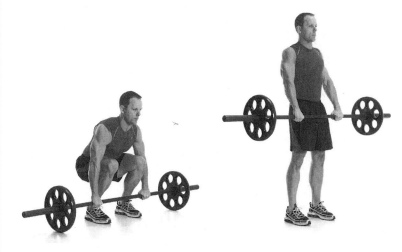

A Place a loaded barbell on the floor, and stand with your feet hip-width apart under the center of the bar. Bend your knees, squat down, and grasp the bar with an overhand grip, with your hands shoulder-width or slightly farther apart.

B Keeping your arms and back straight, extend your knees and hips as you lift the bar and stand. As you lift, keep the bar close to your body. Pull your shoulders back at the top of the lift. Complete 3 sets of 4 to 6 reps.

■ FLAT BARBELL BENCH PRESS

Chest, Shoulders, Triceps

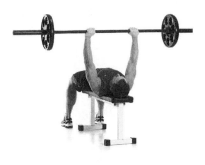 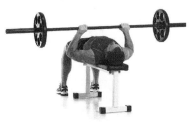

A Lie on a flat bench and position your body so the barbell on the supports is above your face. Grasp the bar with your hands shoulder-width apart. Keep your feet flat on the floor as you lift the weight off the supports and hold the bar above your chest.

B Bend your elbows to the sides as you lower the bar toward your upper chest, stopping when your elbows are in line with your torso.

Pause at the bottom for a second and press back up. Complete 3 sets of 4 to 6 reps.

■ STEPUP
Glutes, Quads, Hamstrings

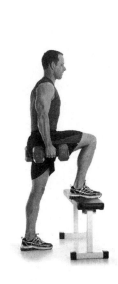

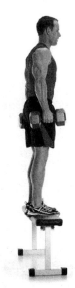

A Holding dumbbells at your sides, stand in front of a weight bench or step that's at least 12 inches high. Place your right foot on top of the bench or step.

B Press into your right foot and extend your right leg as you lift your body over the bench or step. Place your left foot onto the bench or step.

Then step down onto the floor with your right foot. Keeping your torso upright, continue alternating sides until you've stepped up 4 to 6 times on each side. Complete 3 sets.

◼ OVERHEAD BARBELL SHOULDER PRESS

Deltoids, Triceps, Traps

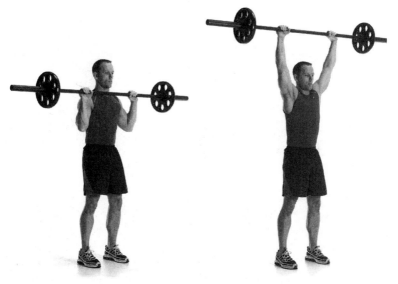

A Grasp a barbell with an overhand grip, with your hands slightly more than shoulder-width apart. Position the bar near your upper chest.

B Press the bar up until your arms are extended overhead.

Lower and repeat, completing 3 sets of 5 to 7 reps.

■ PULLUP
Upper Back, Biceps, Brachialis

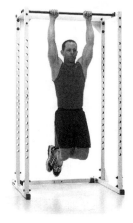

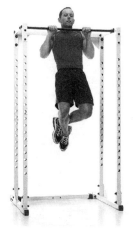

A Hang from an overhead bar with an overhand grip, with your hands shoulder-width apart.

B Pull yourself up until your chin clears the bar. Lower and repeat, completing 5 to 7 reps.

NOTE: If you can't pull up your entire weight, do assisted pullups, either with a partner pushing against your lower back or on a pull-up machine that supports some—but not all—of your body weight.

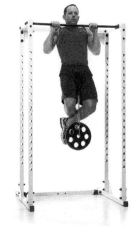

C If you can easily do 5 to 7 reps, either wear a weighted belt or hold a dumbbell between your ankles. Complete 3 sets.

Total-Body Workout #2

■ BARBELL SQUAT
Glutes

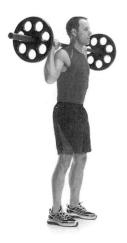 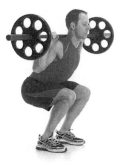

A Position a barbell along the backs of your shoulders, holding the bar with an overhand grip.

B With your body weight equally distributed between your heels and forefeet, bend your knees and bend forward slightly from the hips until your thighs are parallel to the floor.

Then straighten your legs and rise to the starting position. Throughout, keep your head forward, your back straight, and your feet flat on the floor. Complete 3 sets of 4 to 6 reps.

■ DIP

Triceps, Chest

Depending on your strength, you can do this exercise either on a dip bar with or without weight or on a dip/pullup machine that removes some of the weight from your body. If you need added weight, either use a weighted belt or hold a dumbbell between your ankles.

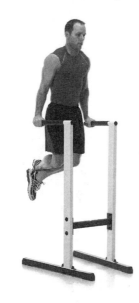

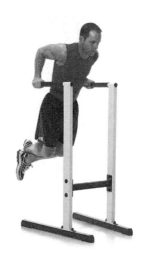

A Mount the dip bar or machine with your palms facing in and your arms extended.

B Keeping your elbows close to your body, bend them and lower your torso until you feel a slight stretch in your shoulders.

Extend your arms and return to the starting position. Complete 3 sets of 4 to 6 reps.

BARBELL GOOD MORNING

Hamstrings, Lower Back

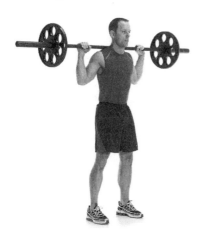
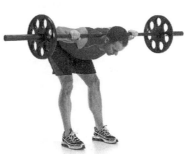

A Position a barbell along the backs of your shoulders, grasping it with an overhand grip, with your hands slightly more than shoulder-width apart.

B Bend forward from the hips as if you were bowing, but keep your back flat (not rounded). Stop when your torso is parallel to the floor.

Keeping your back and knees extended, return to the starting position. Complete 3 sets of 4 to 6 reps.

■ BARBELL CURL
Biceps

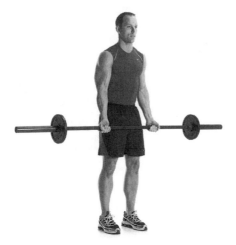

A Grasp a barbell with an underhand grip, with your hands shoulder-width apart and your arms hanging down in front of you.

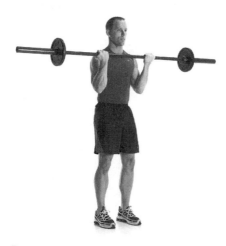

B Keeping your elbows close to your sides, raise the bar until your forearms are vertical.

Lower and repeat 4 to 6 times.
Complete 3 sets.

■ BARBELL ROLLOUT

Abdominals, Lower Back, Shoulders

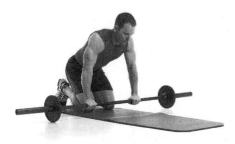

A Kneel on an exercise mat behind a barbell with a 5-pound plate at each end. Grasp the bar with your hands shoulder-width apart and directly beneath your shoulders.

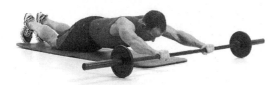

B Slowly allow the bar to roll out and let your body to travel with it. Let your arms extend forward over your head and lower your face as close as possible to the floor without allowing your back to round.

Once you've reached your farthest point, use your core muscles to return to the starting position. Complete 3 sets of 5 to 7 reps.

ENDURANCE-FOCUSED SCHEDULE

Now that you have the moves to help you maximize the workouts you love most, let's talk about how to put it all together. The following weekly schedule works great for people who love cardio but aren't so enthused about the weight room. It includes four cardio sessions and just two weight workouts.

Like the strength-focused schedule earlier in this chapter, it also provides 2 days off. To make up for the extra downtime, you'll add some steady-state exercise to the mix. In this session, do some form of cardio without doing intervals—go out for an easy jog or a bike ride, swim, or hike. Unlike low-intensity cardio, this steady state is official exercise, but you're not pushing it as you would for your interval workouts.

Use the following schedule.

MONDAY: Total-body workout in the morning; interval session in the evening

TUESDAY: 30 minutes of steady-state exercise

WEDNESDAY: Total-body workout in the morning; interval session in the evening

THURSDAY: 30 minutes of steady-state exercise

FRIDAY: Interval session

SATURDAY: Off

SUNDAY: Off

Eating Out on the Plan

Restaurants are where most people's nutrition programs get off track. At home and at work, it's easy to stick to your plan. At restaurants, you encounter a host of decadent choices (including appetizers and desserts). Even when you try to minimize the potential damage and order something you consider safe, you never really know what you're getting, unless you ask.

That's the scary part. The reality is that we all eat out from time to time. Even I do it. I've worked with hundreds of clients who do it. The good news is that you *can* eat out. You can also attend dinner parties, office parties, and birthday parties. You can modify the Metabolism Advantage plan to suit your individual tastes. To do so, ask yourself these questions before you sit down to a meal or snack.

WHERE'S THE COMPLETE PROTEIN?

Metabolism Advantage Rule: Men should eat at least one 6-to-8-ounce serving of complete protein at every meal; women, a 4-ounce serving. A 4-ounce serving is slightly larger than a deck of cards; 8 ounces is two decks. Try to make this protein lean; in other words, take the skin off the chicken or turkey, order lean beef (sirloin is usually the best bet), and stay away from bacon.

WHERE ARE THE VEGGIES?

Metabolism Advantage Rule: You should eat at least two servings (1 to 2 cups per serving) of veggies at every meal or snack. Have them prepared any way you like; just eat them.

WHERE ARE THE CARBS?

Metabolism Advantage Rule: Save nonfruit and nonveggie carbs (pasta, bread, rice, etc.) until after your workout. If you haven't just worked out, don't eat starchy carbs (potatoes or bread), grains (rice, quinoa, pasta), and sugars.

WHERE ARE YOUR FATS COMING FROM?

Metabolism Advantage Rule: You need to consume some fat from animal foods, some from olive oil, some from mixed nuts, some from fish oil, and some from flaxseed oil. You probably won't find fat in the form of flaxseed oil at restaurants and at most dinner parties, but you can take along your fish-oil capsules. Make sure that what you consume at home and away from home adds up to a combination of these good fats. Spread them throughout the day, making sure you get some in each meal.

Providing the correct answers to those questions will help you to create a Metabolism Advantage–worthy meal no matter where you find yourself. If you haven't worked out yet, your meal will consist of lean protein, good fats, and veggies. If you have worked out, you'll eat lean protein, veggies, and a fiber-rich, starchy source of carbohydrate such as quinoa. Follow those rules, and you can't go wrong at any restaurant or party. You can also use them to adapt Metabolism Advantage eating to different ethnicities and food preferences.

For additional help in eating out, follow these pointers.

Avoid caloric drinks. Order water, green tea, or both. Stay away from other drinks, such as sodas, fruit juices, and even coffee with cream and sugar.

Remember the 90 percent rule. Are you breaking any of the Metabolism Advantage rules? If so, count the meal as one of your 10 percent meals that fall outside of the plan and think about how you'll get back on track with the next meal.

Have a backup plan. When looking over a menu, choose two or three meals that may, depending on how they're prepared, follow the Metabolism Advantage rules. Ask the server how each is prepared and what comes on the side. Make special requests (no skin on chicken, for example, or steamed spinach instead of a baked potato) to get the meal to conform to Metabolism Advantage rules. Remember, your meal should be built around protein, have good fats, and include a good amount of vegetables. It should include other carbohydrates only if you have worked out recently.

Add or replace instead of subtract. Don't be afraid to ask that the chef prepare your meal with one or more of the Metafoods discussed in Chapter 3, even if those foods are not already part of the meal. For example, you might ask whether the chef can include mixed nuts or sunflower seeds in your garden salad or prepare it with spinach instead of lettuce. Or you can ask if the restaurant has guacamole or sliced avocado for your salad.

Substitute for carbs. Most restaurant meals contain a protein portion, a carbohydrate portion, and a vegetable portion. If you haven't just exercised, ask to swap the carbohydrate for more protein or vegetables. For example, you might ask for a double serving of grilled asparagus instead of a baked potato or a second chicken breast instead of a serving of pasta.

Go light on the sauces. With the addition of butter during the cooking process (even steaks are prepared with butter to make the meat appear more juicy), sauces to meats, and dressings to salads, the caloric value of a meal can be doubled without increasing the nutritional value at all. Ask if the chef can prepare your meal without additional oil, butter, sauces, or dressings. If you want a little sauce or dressing, ask the server to bring some on the side so that you can use only a small amount.

Spoon on the sauces and dressings. If you want to add sauce or dressing to your meal, do so with a spoon rather than pouring it on from a bowl. While this sounds silly, it works. It's easier to control the amount you add when using a teaspoon. Plus, you'll be a little less zealous with the dressing.

Eating Fast Food

There's gonna come a time when you have to eat, but you don't have a great Metabolism Advantage option available. Don't panic. Instead of throwing your Metabolism Advantage plan out the window, do your best to stick to the rules you just read.

Ask yourself the questions outlined in the eating out section. (Where's the complete protein? Where are the veggies? Where are the carbs? Where are your fats coming from?) To make things easy on you, I went on a fast food quest, searching for foods that meet Metabolism Advantage standards. I actually found quite a few, and I've listed a few of them here. (For more Metabolism Advantage fast food suggestions, go to www.MetabolismAdvantage.com.) Each entry listed for a fast food restaurant represents a complete Metabolism Advantage meal.

WENDY'S

Cup of chili
Mandarin Chicken Salad with Almonds
2 teaspoons of sesame dressing
Cup of ice water
2 fish-oil capsules

MCDONALD'S

Chicken McGrill Sandwich (no mayo; throw out the bun)
California Cobb Salad with Grilled Chicken
2 teaspoons of Low-Fat Balsamic Vinaigrette
Cup of ice water
2 fish-oil capsules

SUBWAY

Grilled Chicken and Baby Spinach Salad
Savory Turkey Breast Wrap
Cup of ice water
2 fish-oil capsules

10

Maintain Your Advantage

The tools you need for a lifetime of metabolism boosting

At this point in your Metabolism Advantage journey, you've either spent 8 weeks eating, exercising, and supplementing according to the Metabolism Advantage rules or spent the past 8 hours sitting in your recliner reading, with a bowl of cheese curls and a beer nearby. If the latter describes you, that's cool. I'm glad you found *The Metabolism Advantage* so compelling. Go ahead and read to the last page. Then get your butt out of that chair, toss the rest of your cheese curls in the trash, and start revving it up.

For the rest of you, however, who have already completed the first 8 weeks (phase 1) of the Metabolism Advantage plan, it's time to ask the all-important question: "What's next?"

As I've mentioned, the plan requires a lifetime commitment to metabolism-boosting eating, exercising, and supplementing. If I could create an 8-week program that fixed everyone's metabolisms permanently, I'd be a very rich man. Alas, such a program does not exist. To maintain your results, you must maintain your focus. That means you must continue to eat right, exercise, and take your supplements. Got that? This isn't the time to start backsliding. Now that you're in the habit of starting the day with eggs, for example, don't celebrate this morning by having a doughnut—or worse—by skipping breakfast entirely. Now that you're in the habit of saving your carbs until after your workout, don't backslide by eating them at any time of day the mood strikes. Now that you're in the habit of filling your plate with the Metafoods, resist the urge to displace those foods with less wholesome choices such as refined bread, pork rinds, and potato chips.

Although you can certainly take a few well-deserved liberties after your 8 weeks of hard work (and you'll find out exactly how to do so in the coming pages), you don't want to slack off so much that you lose traction and slide backward down the slippery slope to where you started: your old sluggish metabolism.

Before I explain how to maintain your results, however, let's take a look at how far you've come. The first 8 weeks of the Metabolism Advantage program really revved up your metabolism up in a big way. If you've been faithful to the program, I have no doubt that you can easily see your results when you look in the mirror. That belly flab? It's either gone or much less noticeable. Those arms? More toned, for sure. You've lost inches of fat off your waist and elsewhere and added lean, calorie-hungry muscle to power your metabolism. Depending on your starting point, you may have lost between 10 and 15 pounds on the scale.

What's more, you're not only leaner but also healthier. If you have blood work done, you'll see improvements in measurements such as total cholesterol levels. Your "good" HDL cholesterol will be higher and your "bad" LDL cholesterol, blood sugar, and triglycerides lower. Your tests will also show improvements in liver function.

Most important, your metabolism has done an about face. You've boosted it by 40 to 60 percent (1,000 to 1,500 calories per day)! Before you started this program, you were fighting a losing battle of eating less and gaining more. It seemed like no matter how little you ate, your belly got pudgier. Now, you're eating the right foods every 2 to 3 hours.

You don't pay attention to portion sizes or calories, yet you're losing fat instead of gaining it! Your co-workers, gym buddies, and friends—who see you eat and eat and eat—keep asking about your hollow leg.

All of that said, if you stop the program right now, you'll lose everything you've worked so hard to build. The unfortunate reality is this: As soon as you stop working out, your metabolism starts slowing down. Even worse, it takes less time to undo the hard work you've completed in the past 8 weeks. If you stop exercising today, your resting metabolism will return to its snail's pace within a few weeks. That body fat? It can come back much faster than it went away.

This holds true whether you stop cold turkey or gradually fall back into your old habits, so right now, make a commitment to yourself to keep it revving. If you stick with the Metabolism Advantage program and follow the advice in this chapter, you'll maintain all the results you've seen so far as well as continue to lose fat until you reach your goal. With each subsequent workout, you'll get even stronger. That means you'll be able to work out harder, increasing the number of calories you burn during exercise.

To do so, however, you have to keep it up. You must continue to eat right, exercise, and take your supplements. Throughout the following pages, you'll find out how to maintain this trinity of a speedy metabolism for a lifetime.

Keep-It-Revving Nutrition

During weeks 1 through 8 of the Metabolism Advantage plan, you followed a set meal plan that laid out not only what to eat but also when to eat it. I did all the planning for you. I even gave you your grocery lists. Now that you've completed phase 1 (the first 8 weeks) of the program, however, it's time for you to become more independent. Although I'm not going to give you a detailed meal plan to follow for the rest of your life, I will give you some simple tools that will make Metabolism Advantage eating simple.

As I've mentioned before, there isn't just one way to eat to boost your metabolism. I hope the past 8 weeks have given you a sample of the kinds of meals and snacks you can eat. If you loved everything presented to you on the meal plans, by all means, go ahead and continue to follow those plans, picking out the days you like best and following them in any order you see fit.

That said, if you are the type of person who needs a little more variety and flexibility, it's time for you to take matters into your own hands. To do so, you'll follow a three-step process. These Metabolism Advantage steps will help you stay on track with your nutrition program no matter where you are eating: at home, at work, or at restaurants. As long as you consistently follow this process, eating well will be a breeze.

NEED MORE METABOLISM ADVANTAGE RECIPES?

What if you grow tired of the recipes included in the Metabolism Advantage eating plan? You can find more convenient and delicious recipes at www.metabolismadvantage.com.

STEP 1: MAKE YOUR METAFOOD QUOTA

As long as you consume three or more servings of Metafoods each week, you can't go wrong.

STEP 2: FOLLOW THE METABOLISM ADVANTAGE MEAL-PLANNING RULES

Make two photocopies of the Metabolism Advantage Meal-Planning Rules on the opposite page. Keep one copy at home and one with you (in your wallet or purse), and consult them when it's time to plan, prepare, or order a meal. Each time you use this guide, you'll reinforce a new, better way of thinking about food. Eventually, you won't have to think about changing your eating habits; the Metabolism Advantage way of eating will become automatic.

THE METABOLISM ADVANTAGE
MEAL-PLANNING RULES

Make sure every meal you eat meets these requirements.

BUILD EACH MEAL AROUND A COMPLETE, LEAN PROTEIN. Make skinless chicken breast, eggs, fish, and lean meat such as ground turkey breast the centerpiece of each meal. Be sure to include salmon, lean red meat, and omega-3 eggs—three of the Metafoods—a few times a week.

EAT VEGGIES AT EVERY MEAL. Veggies balance the acid-producing nature of protein, so eat a big serving of them along with every serving of protein. Maximize your consumption of spinach, tomatoes, and cruciferous vegetables such as broccoli and cauliflower to help meet your Metafood quota.

BALANCE YOUR FATS. You need some fat from animal foods, olive oil, mixed nuts, fish oil, and flaxseed oil. Spread them out throughout the day. When following recipes, check to see whether they have a balance of fats. If a recipe calls for red meat and butter—both sources of saturated fat— consider substituting olive oil for the butter to balance your fat intake. Similarly, when ordering in restaurants, ask the server if you can substitute oil for butter on certain dishes in order to better balance your fat intake.

EAT CARBS AFTER EXERCISE. Save nonfruit and nonveggie carbs (pasta, bread, rice, etc.) until after your workout, when your body will use them most efficiently.

REMEMBER YOUR FISH OIL. Take a capsule or two with each meal and snack.

AVOID CALORIC DRINKS. Drink water, green tea, or both with your meals.

REMEMBER THE 90 PERCENT RULE. Are you breaking any of the above rules? If so, count this meal as one of the 10 percent of your meals that fall outside the Metabolism Advantage guidelines and think about how you'll get back on track with your next meal.

FOOD LABELS 101

Below you'll find a typical example of a food label found on all packaged foods at your local supermarket.

Nutrition Facts

Serving Size
Servings Per Container

Amount Per Serving

Calories 0   Calories from Fat 0

% Daily Value*

Total Fat 0g	**0%**
Saturated Fat 0g	**0%**
Polyunsaturated Fat 0g	
Monounsaturated Fat 0g	
Cholesterol 0mg	**0%**
Sodium 0mg	**0%**
Total Carbohydrate 0g	**0%**
Dietary Fiber 0g	**0%**
Sugars 0g	
Protein 0g	

Vitamin A 0%   •   Vitamin C 0%

Calcium 0%   •   Iron 0%

* Percent Daily Values are based on a 2,000 calorie diet. Your daily values may be higher or lower depending on your calorie needs:

	Calories:	2,000	2,500
Total Fat	Less than	0g	0g
Sat Fat	Less than	0g	0g
Cholesterol	Less than	0mg	0mg
Sodium	Less than	0mg	0mg
Total Carbohydrate		0g	0g
Dietary Fiber		0g	0g

STEP 3: KNOW WHAT YOU'RE EATING

To take your nutritional planning into your own hands, I have two words for you:

1. Food
2. Labels

You must learn how to read food labels. If you don't know what you're eating, you can't know whether you're meeting your Metafood requirements or building your meals around the Metabolism Advantage rules. Once you get comfortable reading food labels, you'll better be able to discriminate among foods. For example, next time you go to the store, pick up a can of pineapple in heavy syrup and check out the grams of sugar listed on the food label. You'll be shocked to see that the manufacturer added 45 grams of sugar to every can! Oops, there goes the food plan, even when you were trying to do your best.

To this end, I've included the following quick primer about what to look for. Consult "Food Labels 101" on the opposite page.

Serving Size. Although you don't need to count calories on the Metabolism Advantage plan, you should still know what you are eating. Many people quickly look at a food's "Calories" listing and mistakenly think they are eating (or drinking) less than they really are. For example, many containers of soft drinks and small packages of snack foods contain two or more servings. When you consume everything in the package in just one sitting, you're getting double or triple the number of calories listed under "Total Calories."

For larger food items, a serving may listed at just four or five chips or crackers, whereas most people eat double or triple that amount. So be careful. You may think that you're getting just 100 calories when you're really getting 300 by eating three times the actual serving size.

Calories. If you follow the Metabolism Advantage rules, use the nutrient-timing rules, and eat from the Metafoods list, your calorie intake should fall right in line. That said, if you are doing all of that and still aren't seeing changes as quickly as you'd like, you might begin examining your total calorie intake to see if that's the problem. You may find that you consistently eat more than you think, particularly when it comes to snack foods.

Total Fat. You want to balance your saturated, polyunsaturated, and monounsaturated fat intake each day, so check out the "Total Fat" listing on food labels to see what fats the food contains.

Total Carbohydrate. This section is important for keeping track of whether you're eating your carbohydrates at the right time of the day. Since you'll be saving most of your nonfruit and nonveggie carbohydrates for after your workouts, make sure this number is relatively low for many of your meals. Although the Metabolism Advantage is *not* a low-carb diet, the plan does require you to save most carbs for when your body needs them most. Unless you've already worked out, watch those sugars closely!

Protein. This simple section tells you how much protein is in a food. Unfortunately, the label doesn't distinguish between complete and incomplete protein, but at least you'll be able to check out how much protein you're getting. Aim for 30 or more grams with each meal.

Ingredients. This is the most important section of your food label. Reading the ingredients list gives you a chance to screen out all the stuff you probably don't want in your body. If you see the following on the list, you probably shouldn't buy the product.

- **High-fructose corn syrup.** This is another name for sugar. Because it's cheap, this sweetener is making its way into just about all packaged foods. From salad dressings to breakfast cereals to snack foods, it's probably in there. High-fructose corn syrup may be even more destructive than sugar because some research shows it may enter the body under the brain's radar. Even though this sweetener contains calories, the brain somehow doesn't sense them—and you end up overeating as a result. I suggest that you never eat the stuff, but if you simply have to (say you have a very strong hankering for a soft drink), at least hold off until after your workout.

- **Glucose-fructose syrup.** This is another form of corn syrup, complete with all of the negative ramifications of high-fructose corn syrup.

- **Partially hydrogenated oil.** Found in margarine and nearly all processed foods, this synthetic fat helps extend the shelf life of foods. Unfortunately, it shortens the shelf life of the human body. Your body has absolutely no use for this synthetic fat. On the contrary, research shows that partially hydrogenated oil is much more dangerous for your heart health than is saturated fat (which, as I've mentioned, is perfectly fine in moderate, balanced amounts). Try to keep your consumption of partially hydrogenated fats (also called trans fats) to zero.

- **Hydrogenated oil.** Minimize your consumption of this fat for the same reasons as partially hydrogenated oils.

- **Any chemical-sounding ingredient.** If you can't pronounce it or find it growing on a plant or in the ground, it's probably not good for you.

Keep-It-Revving Supplements

The Metabolism Advantage supplement plan includes just five supplements. During the past 8 weeks, you've been taking fish oil to rev up your metabolism, protein supplements to support muscle growth and speed metabolism even more, greens supplements to fill in nutritional gaps and alkalinize your body, creatine for overall health and muscle growth, and recovery drinks for postworkout success. Combine those supplements with Metabolism Advantage nutrition that's loaded with micronutrients, antioxidants, and phytochemicals, and you really don't need any more. So if you're following the Metabolism Advantage plan to a T, your needs are probably covered.

That said, over the years I've found that a small number of people with super-sluggish metabolisms could benefit from additional supplementation. How do you know if you're one of these people? Well, if you've followed the Metabolism Advantage plan religiously and noticed only mild results over the past 8 weeks, you can probably benefit from more supplementation for one of two reasons (or possibly both).

1. **Your genes are working against you.** With the human genome project providing insight into the very code that defines who we are, scientists have become aware that when certain genes are present, disease risk is low. With only a subtle alteration in those genes, disease risk can double or triple. In the case of some gene alterations, there's nothing we can do about it. With others, certain nutritional supplements can balance the scales, substantially reducing our risks. The unfortunate reality is that genetically, some people have very slow metabolisms that conserve every single calorie.

2. **You're getting older.** As you age, your cells respond differently. Often, chemicals that promote optimal cellular function and metabolism decrease with age, while chemicals that interfere with optimal function increase with age. Remember the mitochondrion, the powerhouse of the cell, the part where metabolism happens? Well, as you age (or with certain genetic conditions), mitochondria can be damaged by all of those nasty free radicals I discussed earlier. With this mitochondrial damage, the metabolism slows, and cells can actually die. When this happens to skin, it wrinkles and sags. When it happens to

muscles, they shrink and get weak. When it happens to organs, processes like liver detoxification, kidney excretion, and intestinal digestion/absorption suffer. When it happens to your brain, you lose cognitive ability. At what age does this take place? That really depends. Although our birthdays all click by at the same rate, our bodies actually age at different rates. Some 40-year-olds have the cell physiology of 50-year-olds, whereas others have the cell physiology of 25-year-olds.

So if your cells are getting old or your genes are working against you, you may need additional nutrients, especially nutrients that protect your genetic material and your mitochondria. Start with a daily multivitamin/mineral supplement as well as some of the additional supplements listed below. Supplementing with the following nutrients will help power your Metabolism Advantage plan by protecting your mitochondria. For help in finding the best brands of these supplements, go to www.MetabolismAdvantage.com.

Acetyl-l-carnitine. As cells age, levels of a chemical called cardiolipin decrease in the mitochondria. In addition, levels of another chemical, called carnitine, decrease. Both of these chemicals are necessary for optimal mitochondrial structure and fat burning. By supplementing with acetyl-L-carnitine, you improve overall mitochondrial function, in some cases restoring it to youthful levels. To enjoy these benefits, take 2 grams per day.

Alpha lipoic acid (ALA). ALA has many beneficial effects in the body. First, it acts as a powerful antioxidant, defeating those free radicals I keep talking about. Since free radicals can build up in both the fatty parts of your cells (your cell membranes and intracellular lipids) and in the watery parts of your cells (cytosol), you'll need antioxidants that can work under both fatty and watery conditions. ALA is one of the antioxidants that can go both ways. In doing so, it can remove some of the free radicals that other antioxidants like vitamin C (which works in the watery parts) and vitamin E (which works in the fatty parts) can miss. ALA can also improve your tolerance to blood sugar, decreasing your risk of diabetes. When combined with acetyl-L-carnitine, 200 to 300 milligrams of ALA daily can help reduce free radical damage, improve mitochondrial function, improve metabolism, and even improve hearing.

Vitamin C. This antioxidant vitamin repairs and maintains the collagen throughout your body as well as enhancing immunity. Vitamin C in moderate doses (500 milligrams a day) acts as a powerful water-soluble antioxidant, traveling to the watery parts of your cells and neutralizing water-soluble free radicals before they can damage your mitochondria. A healthy, happy mitochondrion leads to a revved-up metabolism.

Vitamin E. Vitamin E in moderate doses (200 IU a day) acts as a powerful fat-soluble antioxidant, traveling to the fatty parts of your cells and neutralizing fat-soluble free radicals before they can damage your mitochondria. As a bonus, vitamin E may also relieve some of the tissue damage caused by intense exercise, helping to reduce post-workout muscle soreness.

Keep-It-Revving Exercise

During the past 8 weeks, you've worked out roughly 5 or more hours a week, 6 days a week, doing relatively intense workouts. You've strengthened each of your major muscle groups by training them with a combination of upper-body, lower-body, and total-body weight-training workouts. You've also mixed in interval exercise a few times each week.

Now it's time to change things up.

During this second phase of the Metabolism Advantage plan—the phase that starts in week 9 and lasts the rest of your life—you have a couple of goals. First, you'll change your exercise program. As I've mentioned, your body adapts to all demands placed upon it. If you do the same type of exercises week after week, your body may adapt to those exercises and your results may plateau, no matter how hard you push yourself. You'll plateau mentally as well. Do the same program week after week, and you get bored. Eventually, you find something else to do rather than go to the gym, and you rev it down rather than up.

For this reason, you did different strength-training routines during weeks 5 through 8 of the Metabolism Advantage plan than you did during weeks 1 through 4. Now, after week 8, you're again ready for a change. It's time to challenge your body and mind with a new set of weightlifting moves. You can accomplish this in a number of ways.

- Cycle through the workouts outlined in weeks 1 through 4, but use heavier weights for each exercise.
- Switch to one of the training programs outlined in Chapter 9.
- Create your own upper-body, lower-body, and total-body workouts using the strategies you've learned in this book, along with the advice available at www.MetabolismAdvantage.com.

In addition to changing the actual exercises, you can also change your weekly program if you prefer. The main Metabolism Advantage workout plan outlined in Chapters 5 and 7 requires six weekly workouts. If you like, you can now scale back your workouts to just 5 days a week—and still keep your metabolism up. (Of course, if you've really enjoyed working out six times a week, you can keep it up and continue to see fantastic benefits.) Both the 5-day-a-week schedule in this chapter (as well as the alternative schedules outlined in Chapter 9) and the 6-day-a-week schedule that you followed during weeks 1 through 8 help build lean, metabolism-boosting muscle. Pick the schedule that works best for you and follow these three golden Metabolism Advantage exercise rules.

1. Strength train each major muscle group at least twice a week. You can accomplish this goal in a number of ways. You might complete just two total-body workouts, or you might do an

upper-body, a lower-body, and a total-body workout. If you love spending time in the weight room, you can even do two upper-body and two lower-body workouts.

2. Complete at least two high-intensity cardio sessions each week. It doesn't matter whether you swim, row, bike, run, or climb stairs as long as you repeatedly alternate between high-intensity (an effort above 7 on a scale of 1 to 10) work intervals and low-intensity recovery intervals.

3. Exercise at least 5 days and 5 hours a week. If your strength-training and intense cardio sessions span just 3 or 4 days, you'll fill in the cracks with low-intensity cardio, such as a walk after work with your spouse, cutting the lawn with a push mower, or actively playing in the yard with your kids or dog. While high-intensity exercise (strength training and intervals) is the best type for improving the way your body looks, feels, and moves, you don't want to overdo it and burn yourself out by completing intense strength-training and cardio sessions most days of the week. High-intensity exercise is demanding on your nervous system. Too much of it can run you down. That's why you want to add a little low-intensity endurance exercise. In addition to helping you meet your 5-hour weekly exercise prescription, low-intensity exercise gives your nervous system a rest, promoting muscle recovery and stress relief.

You can accomplish the three golden rules in a number of ways, and I encourage you to be creative and flexible, coming up with a schedule that suits your personal needs. To give you some help, I've created a 5-day schedule. Just understand that this schedule is just *one* way to do it. It's certainly not the *only way*. If you'd like to schedule your workouts differently, please do! The more you customize your workout schedule to your lifestyle and personal interests, the better your results over the long term.

In the schedule you'll find in the following pages, I've doubled up some of your workouts. On this program, you'll do your interval workouts on the same days as your strength workouts. That gives you 3 days of intense sessions each week. To fill in 2 more days, you'll complete low-intensity cardio.

MONDAY: Lower-body strengthening workout in the morning; interval session in the evening

TUESDAY: 30 minutes of low-intensity exercise

WEDNESDAY: Upper-body strengthening workout in the morning; interval session in the evening

THURSDAY: 30 minutes of low-intensity exercise

FRIDAY: Total-body strengthening workout in the morning; interval session in the evening

SATURDAY: Off

SUNDAY: Off

The Keep-It-Revving Mindset

Now, if you needed to know only what to eat and how to exercise in order to maintain your results for life, everyone would lose weight and keep it off. The sad reality is that all too often, people go on a diet, lose weight, go off the diet, and gain weight. As I've mentioned, this type of on-again-off-again dieting plan ends up slowing your metabolism in the long run.

So you need to take some steps right now to firm up your motivation and stick with the Metabolism Advantage lifestyle. Follow this advice.

Celebrate with a 10 percent meal—then get back on track. If you're the type of person who likes to reflect on your accomplishments, by all means, go ahead and feel pride in your performance. After all, with 8 successful weeks under your belt, you've gotten further in the metabolic battle than most people ever will. Yet there's no resting on your laurels now. You may have won the battle during these past 8 weeks, but now it's time to win the war.

If you absolutely have to, go ahead and celebrate. Have a beer, kick back and watch TV, or do something else that helps you feel good about yourself. Just don't get too carried away.

Don't get me wrong, though. It's pretty hard to undo all of your hard work with one night of intense partying. I'm really not worried about the calories you might consume or the downtime in your exercise regimen. I'm concerned about your mindset.

For most people, a celebration connotes an ending. You celebrate your graduation from high school or college—the end of an era. You celebrate retirement—the end of your work career. This day, however, is not the end. It's a beginning. Yes, be proud of yourself. You've worked hard the past 8 weeks, but you'll work just as hard in the next 8 weeks, and the 8 weeks after that, and the 8 weeks after that. You're going to keep this up for the rest of your life. So be proud, give yourself a pat on the back, and celebrate with a 10 percent meal, but don't be so confident that you feel you can blow it and eat another 10 percent meal tomorrow and the next day and the day after that.

Take a week off from exercise. Even I take a week off every couple of months when I go on vacation or simply want to indulge in a week of rest. This downtime helps my immune system, nervous system, muscles, and brain recover from the intense workouts that I otherwise complete without fail week after week after week. The occasional week off from exercise isn't going to hurt you—in fact, it may even help—assuming you get back on track once the week ends. During your week off, you must eat well, optimizing the Metafoods and building your meals around lean protein and veggies. You'll also need to scale back your portions a little to make up for the calories you're not burning through exercise.

Keep in mind that some people have a hard time getting started again once they've stopped. If you're the type of person who, in the past, has had a hard time making exercise a regular habit, a week off may not be the best thing for you unless it's absolutely necessary.

Respect your body. Until now, you've been on a plan. From here on, however, I want you to think differently about nutrition and exercise. You are not on a plan. This is not an on-or-off proposition. Think of every meal as a chance to do something good for yourself. If you respect your body, you will take every opportunity to do something good for it.

Be realistic. During the past 8 weeks, you made Metabolism Advantage a priority in your life. During the coming weeks and months and years, however, other things may take priority over your Metabolism Advantage lifestyle. Your kid may get sick, causing you to spend your day in a doctor's waiting room and erasing the time you would have spent in the gym. You may have a big project at work, causing you to work 12-hour days for a week or two. In other words, you will have some perfect Metabolism Advantage days along with some imperfect ones. That's cool. Just keep moving forward to the best of your ability most of the time. Revving it up and keeping it revved up isn't a black-and-white situation. If you miss one workout or don't eat as perfectly as you'd like, you won't lose it all. It's okay if you don't stick to Metabolism Advantage principles 100 percent of the time. Ninety percent of the time is all I'm asking of you.

Remember the 90 percent rule I discussed earlier. With both your exercise and nutrition, you don't need 100 percent perfection; 90 percent adherence to the program is still an A.

Be prepared for all challenges and difficulties. Throughout the pages of *The Metabolism Advantage*, you found the workouts and nutritional recommendations to follow on a perfect day. You will have more imperfect days than perfect ones. On these days, try to stick with at least two of the three pillars of the Metabolism Advantage plan. If you don't have time to exercise, for example, try to eat well and take your supplements. If you can't possibly manage to eat well, at least fit in your workout and take your fish oil.

Also, be creative. Let's say your boss asks you to work late every day during the week. What do you do? Maybe, instead of having five intense workouts, you religiously fit in your two weight-training workouts and instead of the interval sessions, you walk during your lunch break. You order your lunch from a restaurant—one that serves lean protein and veggies—and eat at your desk. You have a Super Shake for dinner. You do what you can.

Revisit your goals. Remember the ones you set in Chapter 6? How are you doing? If you've already reached some short-term goals, go ahead and set some more. There's nothing like a goal on the horizon to keep you motivated.

Continue to monitor your progress. Keep Metafood checklists to help you stay on track. Mark down how well you are doing nutritionally—such self-monitoring will help you see in black and white precisely how well you are sticking to the Metabolism Advantage principles. Are you following them 90 percent of the time? Eighty percent of the time? Fifty percent of the time? Your checklists won't lie.

If you haven't done so already, join an exercise community. This "community" can come in many forms. It may be the other folks in the weight room at the gym. It may consist of a couple guys at work who share similar fitness and nutrition goals. Or it may consist of a running partner or a spouse who walks with you after work. It doesn't matter what form your community takes as long as you have one. These people will help keep you motivated, help you surmount bumps along the road ahead, and help support your progress.

A Lifetime of Revving It Up

Throughout the pages of this book, you've learned many important lessons about what revs up and what slows down your metabolism. The Metabolism Advantage principles that you have learned in this chapter allow you to stay on the program without following a set plan. That's the last principle for a lifetime of success on this program: Be flexible. To continue to rev up your metabolism, you don't need a "program" to follow. What you need is to make sure you're adhering to Metabolism Advantage principles at least 90 percent of the time, day in and day out.

Rather than mindlessly following a set of directions that someone else has drawn up for you, this more flexible approach allows *you* to pick the destination and find the route that best fits your needs and interests. I've provided the map for you, but you, based on your lifestyle, will find the best route from point A to point B. For some people, that's the highway. For others, it's the back roads. And for still others, it's a combination of both. You still arrive at point B, but you get there in the most enjoyable and least stressful way possible.

If you hit any potholes or suffer any flat tires along the way, don't abandon your car on the side of the road. Rather, go to www. MetabolismAdvantage.com. Think of it as a global positioning system for your body. I designed this site to provide you with inspiration, information, and motivation to support you all the way through and beyond your 8-week Metabolism Advantage transformation.

You've come a long way, but you also have a long way to go. Wave good-bye to those old metabolism-slowing habits and embrace the metabolism-boosting habits you've learned during the past 8 weeks. I wish you much success.

Conversion Chart

These equivalents have been slightly rounded to make measuring easier.

VOLUME MEASUREMENTS			WEIGHT MEASUREMENTS		LENGTH MEASUREMENTS	
U.S.	*Imperial*	*Metric*	*U.S.*	*Metric*	*U.S.*	*Metric*
¼ tsp	–	1 ml	1 oz	30 g	¼"	0.6 cm
½ tsp	–	2 ml	2 oz	60 g	½"	1.25 cm
1 tsp	–	5 ml	4 oz (¼ lb)	115 g	1"	2.5 cm
1 Tbsp	–	15 ml	5 oz (⅓ lb)	145 g	2"	5 cm
2 Tbsp (1 oz)	1 fl oz	30 ml	6 oz	170 g	4"	11 cm
¼ cup (2 oz)	2 fl oz	60 ml	7 oz	200 g	6"	15 cm
⅓ cup (3 oz)	3 fl oz	80 ml	8 oz (½ lb)	230 g	8"	20 cm
½ cup (4 oz)	4 fl oz	120 ml	10 oz	285 g	10"	25 cm
⅔ cup (5 oz)	5 fl oz	160 ml	12 oz (¾ lb)	340 g	12" (1')	30 cm
¾ cup (6 oz)	6 fl oz	180 ml	14 oz	400 g		
1 cup (8 oz)	8 fl oz	240 ml	16 oz (1 lb)	455 g		
			2.2 lb	1 kg		

PAN SIZES		TEMPERATURES		
U.S.	*Metric*	*Fahrenheit*	*Centigrade*	*Gas*
8" cake pan	20 × 4 cm sandwich or cake tin	140°	60°	–
9" cake pan	23 × 3.5 cm sandwich or cake tin	160°	70°	–
11" × 7" baking pan	28 × 18 cm baking tin	180°	80°	–
13" × 9" baking pan	32.5 × 23 cm baking tin	225°	105°	¼
15" × 10" baking pan	38 × 25.5 cm baking tin	250°	120°	½
	(Swiss roll tin)	275°	135°	1
1½ qt baking dish	1.5 liter baking dish	300°	150°	2
2 qt baking dish	2 liter baking dish	325°	160°	3
2 qt rectangular baking dish	30 × 19 cm baking dish	350°	180°	4
9" pie plate	22 × 4 or 23 × 4 cm pie plate	375°	190°	5
7" or 8" springform pan	18 or 20 cm springform or	400°	200°	6
	loose-bottom cake tin	425°	220°	7
9" × 5" loaf pan	23 × 13 cm or 2 lb narrow	450°	230°	8
	loaf tin or pâté tin	475°	245°	9
		500°	260°	–

Index

Underscored page references indicate boxed text and charts.
Boldface references indicate illustrations.

R

Recipes, 165–66, <u>352.</u> *See also specific foods*
Recordkeeping, for workouts, 207. *See also specific workouts*
Recovery, after workouts, 92–93, 98, 135
Recovery drinks, postworkout, 69, 86–88
Restaurant dining guidelines, 344–47
Resting metabolic rate (RMR), 15
 factors increasing, <u>27</u>, **27**, <u>36</u>, **36**, 92
 factors reducing, <u>19</u>, **19**, 45, 46
Rice
 Fajita Chicken and Rice, 187
Rice protein supplements, 80–81
RMR. *See* Resting metabolic rate

S

Salad dressings
 controlling amount of, 347
 Flax Your Dressing, 182–83
 I Love Olive, 182
Salads
 Carrot Salad, 178
 chopping vegetables for, 174
 Fruit Salad, 178
 Mediterranean Salad, 176
 Metabolism Advantage Salad, 175
 Metabolism Advantage Tabbouleh, 181
 Mixed-Bean Salad, 180
 Toasted Quinoa Salad, 176–77
Salmon
 as Metafood, 64
 Pecan-Crusted Salmon, 194
 Rosemary Salmon and Asparagus on the Grill, 192
 Salmon Burger Stroganoff, 191
 Salmon in Basil Cream Sauce, 193
Sauces, with restaurant meals, 347

Scallions
 Metabolism Advantage Tabbouleh, 181
Scallops
 Almond-Crusted Sea Scallops with Tomato-Onion Gratin, 196
 Seared Scallops in Spinach Cream Sauce, 197
Serving size, on food labels, 355
Shopping lists, for Metabolism Advantage planner, 208–9, 216–17, 224–25, 232–33, 240–41, 248–49, 256–57, 264–65
Snacks
 Chocolate Peanut Butter Bar, 203
 No-Bake Strawberry Cheesecake, 202–3
Social support for change, assessing, 145, 153–55
Spinach
 Greek Omelet, 167
 Metabolism Advantage Salad, 175
 as Metafood, 64
 Scrambled Eggs and Greens, 169
 Seared Scallops in Spinach Cream Sauce, 197
 Spinach and Cheese Omelet, 168
 Spinach Sauté, 175
Squash
 Citrus Chicken–Stuffed Acorn Squash, 185
Strawberries
 Fruit Salad, 178
 No-Bake Strawberry Cheesecake, 202–3
Strength-focused workouts
 lower-body high-repetition, weeks 1-4
  barbell hack squat, 294, **294**
  Bulgarian split squats with dumbbells, 292, **292**
  lying leg curl, 295, **295**
  suitcase deadlift, 293, **293**

V

Vegetables. *See also* Salads; *specific vegetables*
 benefits from, 53–58
 chopping, 174
 cruciferous, 64–65
 in greens supplements, 82–84
 inadequate intake of, 82
 in restaurant meals, 345
 when to eat, 67–68, <u>353</u>
Vitamin C, 360
Vitamin E, 360
Vitamins and minerals, importance of, 32–33
VO₂ max, increasing, 136

W

Web site. *See* Metabolism Advantage Web site
Weight loss, protein improving, 53
Weight regain, from diets, 45–47
Wheat berries
 Roasted Chicken with Rosemary Wheat Berries, 186
Workout times, sample meals for, 70–73

Y

Yams
 Baked Yam and Turkey Meatball Marinara, 190
Yogurt, 64

Metabolism Advantage Readers: Where to next?

Don't close the book on your progress! Get 24/7 support online at:

www.MetabolismAdvantage.com

For years, I've been helping my own personal clients using a private, invitation-only online support forum—a password-protected Web site where you can ask questions, get answers, seek and provide help, and get support from like-minded people pursuing the same goals as you.

Well, here's your invitation to join the club!

Why would you want to join?

- **Get help and support from coaches and fellow members, 24/7.** Ask questions and get answers, wherever you are, whenever you like.

- **Get access to exclusive articles by me,** where I'll translate the latest research into plain-language strategies you can actually use to better your physique.

- **Learn how to perform the exercises using our online video database**—you'll know more than 99 percent of the members at your gym!

- **Build on what you've learned in *The Metabolism Advantage*.** We'll point you to tons of resources to take you through these 8 weeks and beyond.

And there's more—including some very cool members'-only projects that I'm working on as we go to press.

Here's the best part: It's free! Consider it my thanks for buying this book. All I ask is that you keep it quiet—remember, this is for customers only.

To continue your progress and take advantage of all the site has to offer, join now at: www.MetabolismAdvantage.com

See you online!

[signature]

John M. Berardi, PhD, CSCS

PS: You'll need to enter a special username and password the first time you go to the site. That'll take you to the secret signup page, where you can create an account of your own. Here's what to enter:

Username: **guest**
Password: **metabolism**

---

member LOGIN

Username:
guest

Password:
metabolism

Login

Forgot your password?

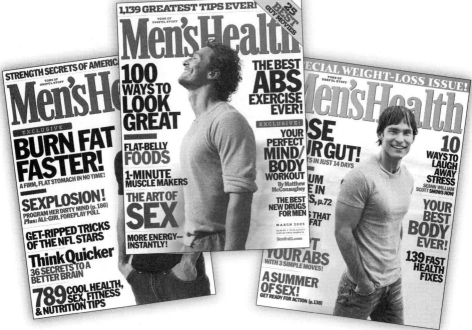
200562202

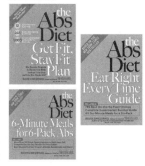
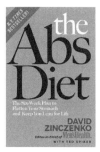

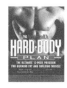